MALABAR FLAVORS

Timeless Memories *of* Nurturing Recipes

Daisy Kuchinad, M.D.

Copyright © 2019 by Dr. Daisy Kuchinad, M.D

All rights reserved. This book or any portion thereof may not be reproduced or used in any manner whatsoever without the express written permission of the publisher except for the use of brief quotations in a book review.

Editors: Ketan Kuchinad & Patricia Conover

Cover & interior design: Islam Farid

ISBN: 978-1-7341822-1-7

www.ahimsaretreats.com

DEDICATION

This book is dedicated to:

My grandparents and elders whose way of life is rooted deep in my consciousness.

My parents, Anna and Varkey, who had the courage to come across the world so that their children could dream bigger.

My children, Ketan and Kamini, who courageously supported me through difficult times.

My husband, Chet, whose sustained support made this journey possible.

And to Swaran Masi, my adopted mother, who keeps me on track.

TABLE OF CONTENTS

- Dedication — 3
- Table of Contents — 4
- Preface — 7

EARLIEST MEMORIES — 17

- Spiced Mashed Tapioca — 18
- Banana Leaf Wrapped Baked Fish Roe — 24
- Grandma's Shrimp Curry & Steamed Shrimp — 30
- Crepes Roasted in Banana Leaf — 38

BREAKFAST — 43

- Miriam and Mali's Cashew and Raisin Oatmeal — 44
- Mali and Miriam's Sweet & Savory Vegetable Roasted Cream of Wheat — 50
- Coconut Stuffed Birds Nest Rice Noodles — 54

BREAKFAST, BRUNCH AND OTHER MEALS — 61

- Kerala Classic Fermented Rice Crepes — 62
- Rice and Lentil Crepes and Buns — 70

CURRIES AND LENTILS — 79

- Grandma's Sunday Egg Roast Curry — 80
- Kerala Style Coconut Flavored Dal — 84

VEGETABLES — 91

- Raw Sautéed Papaya — 92
- Grandma's Chinese String Bean Sauté — 96
- Mung Dal Stir Fry — 100
- Aunt Lily's Sautéed Brown Beans — 104
- Spiced Mashed Potatoes — 110

YOGURT DISHES — 115

- Golden Spiced Buttermilk — 116
- Mali's Konkani Yogurt Rice — 120
- Mali and Miriam's Yogurt Dishes — 126

SNACKS — 133

- Jackfruit Flavored Rice Cakes — 134
- Plantain Fritters — 140
- Grandma's Overripe Banana Fritters — 146

FLAT BREADS — 151

- Whole Wheat Flat Breads — 152

CHUTNEYS, SAMBAR & GINGER RELISH — 157

- Ginger Relish — 160
- Coconut and Mint Chutneys — 162
- Sambar — 163

The Story of Ahimsa — 165

The Spice Wheel — 176

Glossary — 178

PREFACE

Life Energy

The ancient sages tell us that all of the manifest world is a dynamic energy, folded into different forms. It is an illusion of the senses. Modern quantum physics confirms that there is no "matter" per se, only energy vibrating at certain frequencies that give the impression of being something more concrete. Both of these statements appear to say the same thing using different words.

What is Energy?

Energy is the entity which causes change. Energy creates and destroys, brings into existence, and removes from existence the illusion of what we consider "matter" or "reality." Ancient sages and modern scientists alike have postulated that everything in the created universe emanates from one unified energy field, and that, ultimately, it is a zero-sum game. All energies belong to the same unified whole and are intrinsically connected. Nonetheless, in order for the universe to exist in its current state of dynamism, energy must be constantly bartered and exchanged, thereby causing an ongoing manifestation of reality. The energy of each manifested entity, whether it is animate or inanimate, is being continuously modulated and shaped by intrinsic and extrinsic energy dynamics. This means that our internal and external environment is constantly molding our energy. People, animals, trees, water, air, the food that we choose to put into our bodies, and even our thoughts and emotions all impact our very essence by determining the quantity and quality of energy that we experience and exude. Moreover, and in accordance with the principle known as the "observer effect," the energy we direct at ourselves, at others, and at the world around us, unequivocally causes an energy shift in the very subject or object of our intention. This is remarkable!

As such, we must become more conscious of the way in which we treat, handle and give of our vital selves, for that very essence of who we are is simply too precious to misuse or waste. This book is, in principle, a treatise on the impact that our diet has and the role that it plays in determining the nature of our life energy. Consuming food is one of the most prominent, dominant, and conscious energy transactions taking place between us and the world in which we live each and every day. It is a life sustaining activity that we engage in repeatedly and one in which free will plays a vital and critical role. Thus, the foods we choose to eat, the methods and intentions with which we prepare them, and the ways in which we choose to eat those foods play a pivotal role in the quality and meaning of our lives. In a very palpable and literal sense, we become both what we eat and how we eat it!

It is my hope and wish that, through the writing of these words, I will succeed in exposing the spiritual, psychological and intangible role that food and the ways in which we commune with it influence our lives.

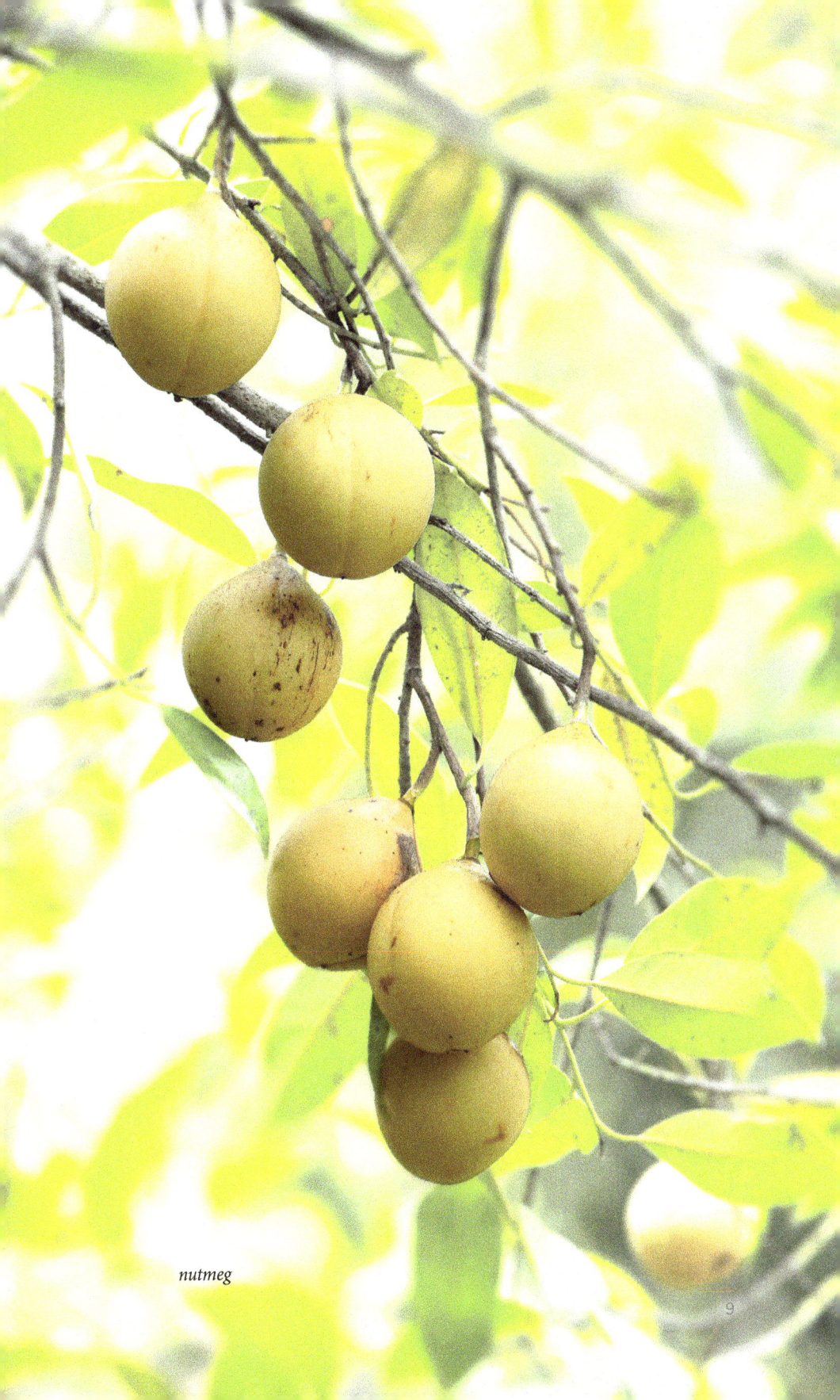
nutmeg

Introduction

In each of the seventeen years I spent growing up in India, the two months of summer vacation were highlighted by our family trip to our ancestral homes in Kerala. In order to get to these homes, which are situated about 2000 kilometers south of where we lived in northern India, my two brothers, my aunt, and I would travel for three days and nights by train. We looked forward to this trek with such delight and anticipation that our preparations began well in advance. Numerous adventures came our way as the steam engine roared and sputtered down to the south, passing through the arid lands of Madhya Pradesh, the parched deserts of Andhra Pradesh, and the lush green mountains and forests of the Deccan mountain ranges before finally coming to rest on that sliver of land known as Kerala, which is nestled within the southwestern coastline of India.

The name "Kerala" means "The Land of Coconuts" and is also known historically as the Malabar Coast. This is the same land that spice traders in ancient times traversed as they made their way along the Silk Road and over the Arabian Sea. None other than Christopher Columbus set forth on his epic voyage to find the exotic spices of this place and lost his way, stumbling upon a different New World. It is in this brave new world that I now reside, struggling and striving to keep the memories alive while fervently hoping to transmit the wisdom and importance of a viable, sustainable, and life-affirming way of eating that is so valuable yet so quickly disappearing from our midst.

My father's family hailed from the area located in the backwaters of Kerala, and my mother's, from the mountainous terrain at the tail end of the Deccan ranges. These two oases were located just a few kilometers away from each other, and our entourage of young cousins would gather in one or the other home, spending eight sun-drenched weeks each year, frolicking and enjoying days of heavenly abandon in the ancestral homes. We would go fishing and canoeing, pick mangoes and custard apples, suck the nectar out of banana and hibiscus flowers, all while exploring with wide-eyed curiosity these seemingly endless, sprawling and fascinating vistas. The most memorable moments of these unrestrained days revolved around the events taking place near my paternal grandmother's hearth, where meals and snacks appeared as our hunger demanded and where Grandma and her brood of daughters and daughter-in-laws seemed to take incomparable pleasure in creating our next, special treat. Most of the recipes in this book come from a desire to rekindle and actualize the most vivid and joyful of these memories—the memories that bring me back, over and over again, to these magical places with a craving to recreate the same tastes, textures, aromas, and way of caring for one another. The memories are brought to life by traditions that mean sharing something purposeful and are a way of nurturing and passing on the meaning of life.

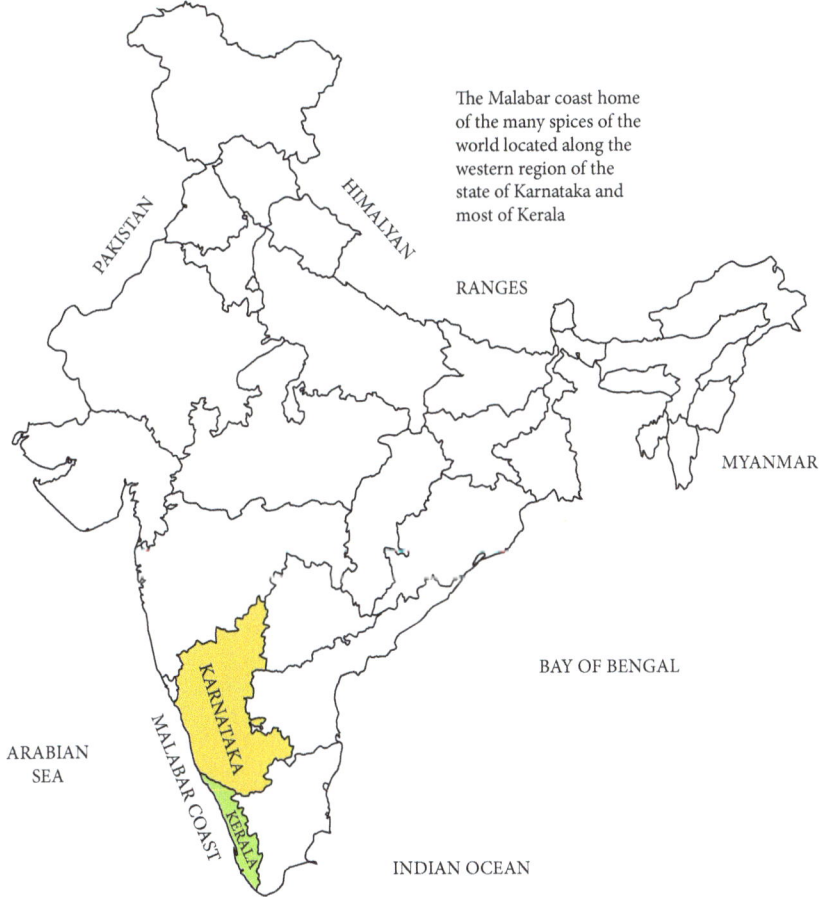

Though we cannot create the same surroundings and context, we can attempt to create new ones that cradle the gift of caring and craft. With the inexorable march of time, Kerala itself has changed dramatically, abandoning old traditions and customs and now resemble the New World more and more every day. Streets clogged with cars, mega-grocery stores and Western-style bakeries where everything is weighed, packaged and shelved, spring up every few yards while the pantries and kitchens of yesteryear remain bare. The diaspora has caused people to migrate far and wide. Yet despite the distance, both physical and interpersonal, attempts are constantly made to carry these tastes and smells along with these travelers to far-flung and foreign lands. In fact, every city in America can boast of well-stocked, Indian grocery stores, where every imaginable ingredient is available, albeit packed and shelved for months, and often having lost the life essence that, in the past, held the secrets of transformation.

Many of these wanderers seem confused but can only resign themselves to the fact that these same ingredients do not bring them the joy they once did. The strings that tethered families together are slowly but surely melting away; caring and craft have been replaced with convenience and appearance. It is much easier to reserve a seat at the local restaurant, when, at the end of the meal, each person can return to his or her cozy sofa and bed. There, with a flick of a button, one can escape into the two-dimensional, virtual world of effortless love and comfort while the food in the belly churns and lurches about, looking for integration, failing to do so and, instead, only intensifying the loneliness, heartache and producing heartburn.

This book is an attempt to weave precious people and their cherished stories into the activities that we do, to connect the beauty, wholeness and alchemy of yesterday's family unit with the disparate shards that remain today. It is hoped that the anecdotes featured in this book—ones of hope, love, nurture and sustenance, of unbreakable bonds and shared chemistry, and ones infused with a treasure trove of opportunities to reconnect with the sturdiness and stability of a time gone by—will motivate and encourage the reader to be on the lookout for new and creative ways of forging a more lasting, meaningful, and purposeful existence of one's own. It is time for our relationship with our food, with one another, and with the world we live in, to move from transactional to transformational. It is time to consciously shift from spending our days counting calories and analyzing protein content, and skipping from one fad to another in search of that elusive formula we are told will produce the superman or woman of our fantasies, to what is real, lasting and sustainable. The true artistry that goes into making food nourishing and nurturing is inextricably connected to the motivation, love and caring associated with that meal's preparation. The intimacy imparted to each dish gives rise to a genuine and heartfelt level of sharing, camaraderie, companionship and communion.

The natural outcome of such deep bonding is the validation each person feels and the impartation of the message that our lives matter, that we truly rely on each other. When all of us—family, friends, —sit together and partake of a meal, we are sharing life energy, sustaining ourselves while effortlessly sending a message of love and caring to each being around us. The food itself, a product of sacrifice and dedication, absorbs this message, sending waves of healing and inspiring energy back into our bodies and souls, to be used as fuel for physical and metaphysical well-being.

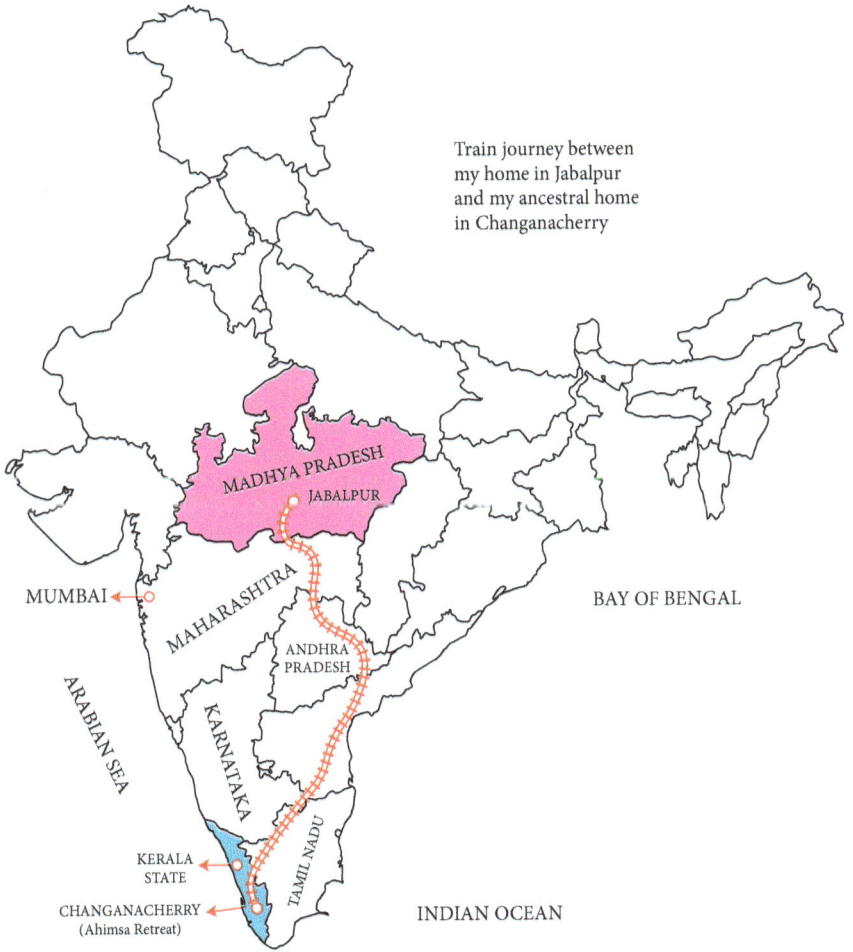

There are those among us who have to come to the realization that sharing a meal is in fact a transformational experience, one might even say, a holy communion. What we eat, how we eat and where we eat will determine how our bodies and minds will feel and behave. Even the healthiest meal, eaten alone, does not nourish the body and soul like a shared meal prepared by someone you know, love and trust, and who you believe put in a great deal of effort and intention. When food is prepared with a desire to please and comfort, then the experience of eating that food has the ability to change and transform the one with whom it is shared. Such an elevated activity promotes cooperation, inspiration, creativity, and counseling and often leads to the sharing of victories, failures, joys, sorrows and ways of arriving at needed solutions to troubling problems. The possibilities are limitless when what we ingest, how we create and share it, who we eat with, and where we are when we do so, are done in service to this higher notion of transformation and holistic growth.

In today's demystifying, sterile and shallow society, we live in communities where a single person or, at most, a couple, luxuriates in supremely comfortable surroundings, occupying pristinely kept homes, with spotless kitchen counters, that one enters mostly to heat a prepared meal in the microwave. The cabinets of these kitchens patiently wait to be opened, their sparkling utensils, neatly stacked away in compartments, often remaining unseen and unused for weeks and months at a time. All the while, this person settles, day after day, for a sandwich containing cold, prepared ingredients that are slapped together so as to fulfill the caloric needs of the person, yet completely and abysmally failing to nourish. The body aches and the soul pines, yet the pain of isolation and the loneliness only grow, culminating in the feeling of being unloved and that one's life simply does not matter.

We as a species need to make it acceptable and desirable to have well-used, messy kitchen counters. We must welcome, with great fanfare, the occasional whiff of exotic cooking emanating from a neighbor's home during a holiday or family celebration. We must learn to love the scent of all that is good, wholesome and satisfying flowing into the hallways and challenging and surprising our noses. We must get used to knocking on a sick neighbor's door, unannounced, to offer a bowl of homemade soup, good bread and a helping of compassion. And we must compel ourselves to knock on a neighbor's door if we ourselves are sick and in need of help.

This book ends with the story of the Ahimsa Gardens. The word "Ahimsa" means 'non-violence". Most of the photographs of flora and fauna featured in this book comes from Ahimsa Gardens. This garden which showcases medicinal plants and rare and endangered trees was born out of an attempt to rescue the land on which the garden sits from being quarried. This garden also showcases environmental sustainability principles such as rainwater harvesting, natural fertilizers, pesticides and traditional cultivating practices. Many of the vignettes in the book take place in and around Ahimsa Gardens which is my home and retreat in India.

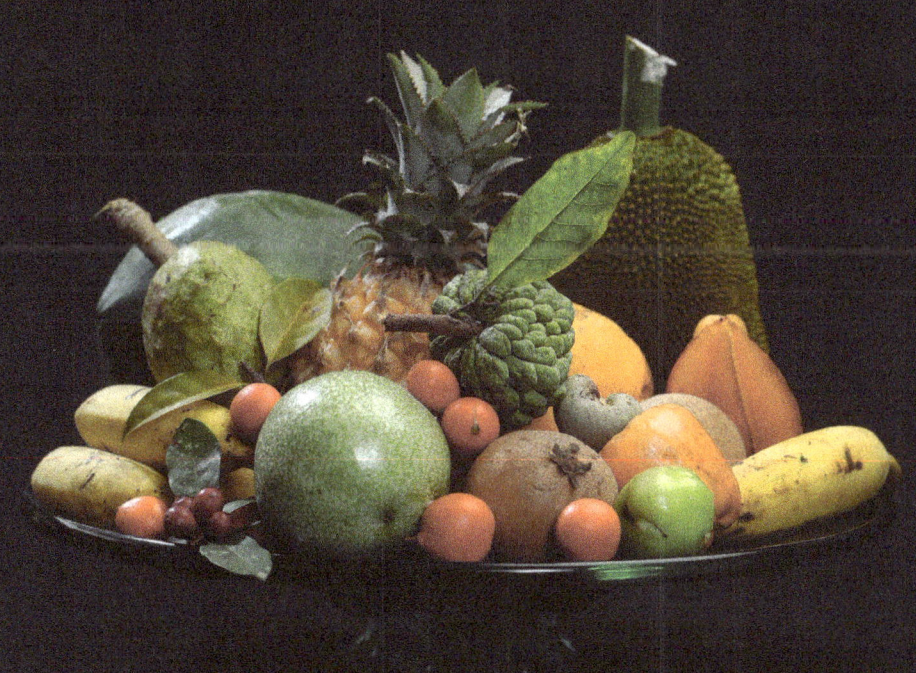

Fruits from Ahimsa Garden

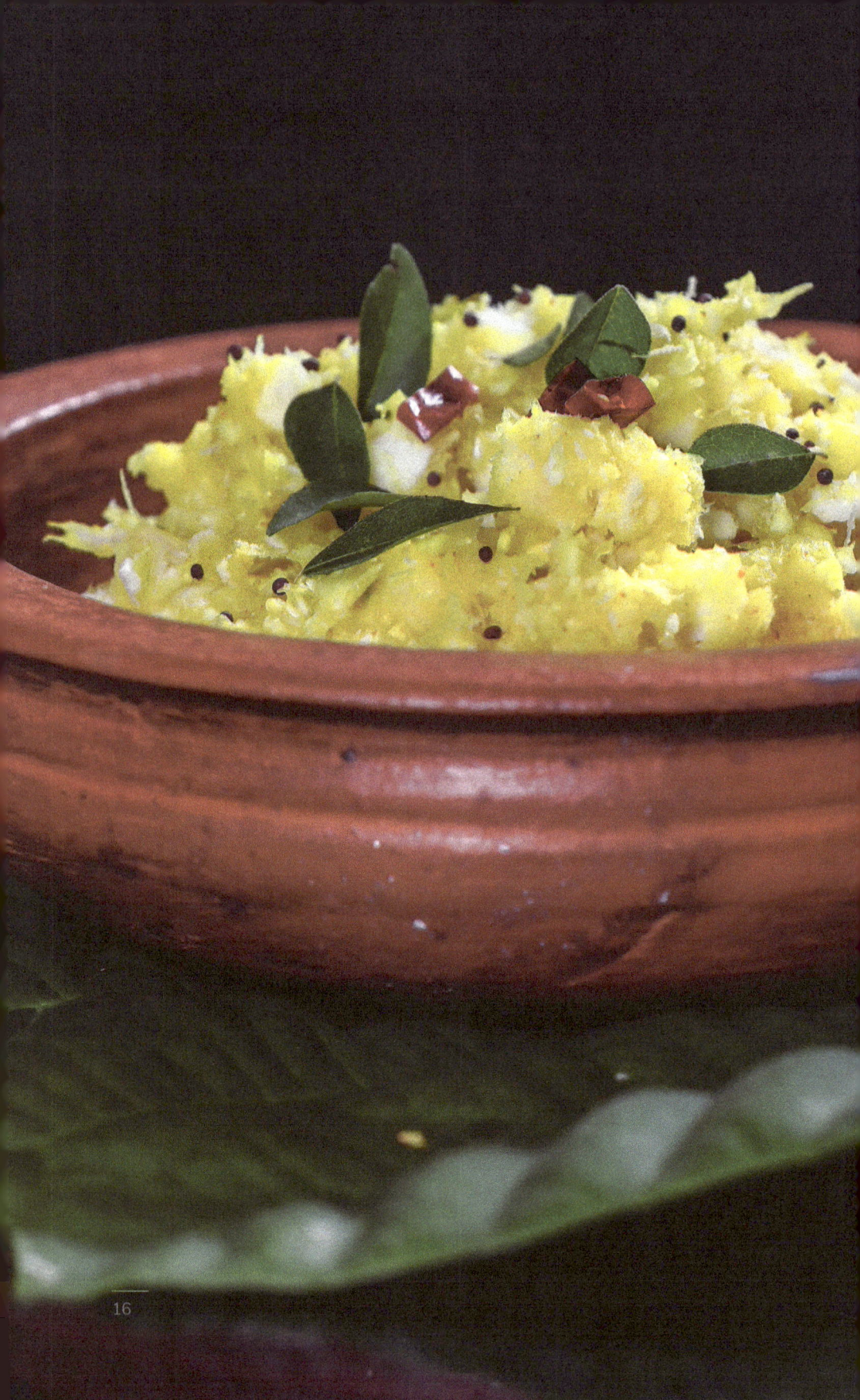

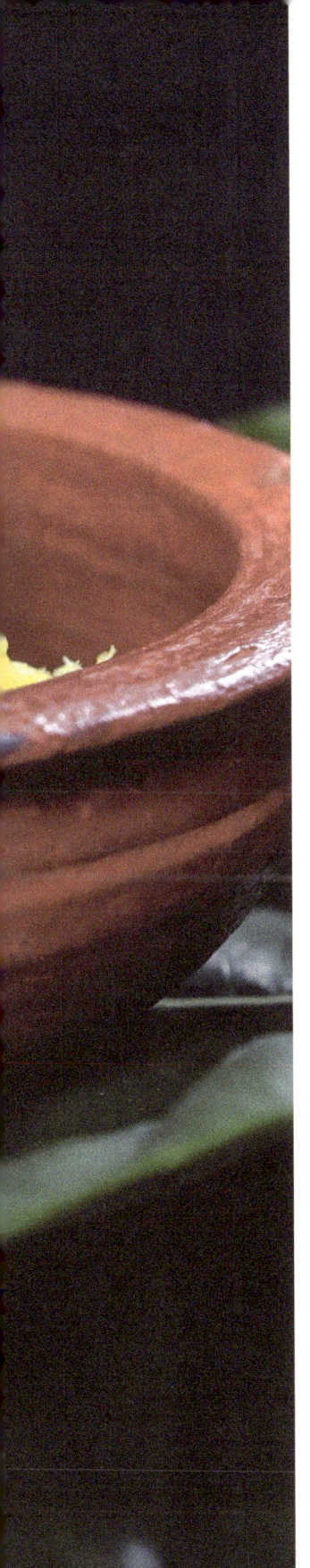

EARLIEST MEMORIES

SPICED MASHED TAPIOCA
Kappa Veakichhade

My childhood summer vacations were spent in two homes, and the events that took place during those tranquil years have become the fondest memories of my life.

The first of the two, my maternal ancestral home, is located at the tail end of the southwestern mountain ranges of India, known as the Deccan Heights. This region is considered to be one of the most biodiverse places on the planet, second only to the Amazon Basin. The second, my father's ancestral home, is in the same general region, known as the Backwaters, located in the flatlands at or below sea level in some places, about fifteen kilometers away.

One of my childhood memories is being carried on the shoulders of my father or an uncle as they traveled over many kilometers of dusty, hilly back roads, to my mother's ancestral home. The first half of the journey through the backwaters took about two hours in one of grandpa's home made canoes. Sitting on a wooden plank seat built into one end of the canoe, I would take great pleasure in letting the fingers of one hand glide over the cool waters while the other hand held tightly to the seat. Patches of white and pink water lilies and water hyacinth, with their complex bluish-purple flowers, watched silently as the canoe drifted noiselessly along its course. Once in a while, I would beg the adult rowing the boat to pick a lily that was too beautiful to resist, and I would hold onto it like a treasure, admiring its stunning design and colors throughout the rest of the way.

Fruit-laden banana, coconut, mango, jackfruit, and papaya trees stood grandly on the banks, piquing my curiosity and awe as we made our way through the meandering streams, rivers and seasonally-flooded paddy fields. Sometimes we delighted in an unexpected snack from low lying branches of mango trees, laden with ripe fruit and inviting us to pick and taste. The fruit was washed in the then-sparkling river water and handed over for their delicious, succulent pulp to be sucked directly out of their leathery sacs. Women washing clothes or dishes or bathing their young children at the steps to the water added to the pageantry of this tantalizing vision.

Once we got to the boat jetty in Changanacherry and tethered the canoe to a nearby tree or post, the remainder of our odyssey was very often on foot. Bus service was sporadic and infrequent at best, and taxis, rickshaws and other modes of transportation were rare and unaffordable at that time.

> *During my childhood I was known to be frail, with poor agility, often falling and scraping my knees with the slightest misstep. The elders preferred to carry me on their shoulders than deal with the frequent falling and first aid.*
>
> *Holding tightly to my father or uncle's forehead, I soaked in all the sights and sounds of the surroundings, pretending and dreaming as much as I wanted. I felt secure, special and loved, almost like a princess in the fairy tales that my father told me at bed time during the few precious days we had during summer vacation.*
>
> *During these very young years, I saw my father and mother only twice a year, for a month at a time, when they were stationed in the army in Northern India in two different locations. During these very special times, I was clearly the center of my father's attention and relished the times we had together on our special evening dates. After the afternoon siesta, evening tea, and a cool bath in the stream in front of the ancestral home, my face and body sprinkled with Ponds talcum powder, we set forth on one of our intimate evening walks. My lithe frame hoisted high on his strong shoulders and crisscrossing the narrow paths of the paddy fields, we remained out until late evening.*
>
> *The events during one of these evening walks would touch my soul and transform me permanently. I was about five, my gaze piercing the distant horizon, the sky a salmon pink and the breeze pregnant with the rhythms of the devotional music from the faraway Hindu temples. This music, to this day, leaves me with a sweet, primordial feeling of*

melancholy. I remember my father reassuring me, "You know you are my princess and there is nothing in this world you cannot do if you put your mind to it." Now, more than half a century later, whenever I doubt myself, his words resonate reassuringly, and I cannot help but smile as I recollect the love that kept me strong. The bond that was formed and the lessons he taught me, even at a very young age, will remain indelibly etched in the recesses of my soul and remain my safe harbor for my journey through this life.

On the tail end of the journey to my maternal home, we got off the main roads. As we started tracking the smaller, gravel-strewn roads of the rolling hills and heading toward the low-roofed traditional Keralan homes that blended into the lush greenery, we would be welcomed by patches of well-tended rows of tapioca plants. Growing from single golden stems, and standing on small mounds of earth, their finger-like leaves would fan out in all directions, resembling hands attached to slender forearms inviting us home.

As the plants matured, shooting up as much as five to seven feet in height, the roots would mature underground, producing fleshy, sweet-potato-like tubers. Inside the outer leathery, pinkish-brown skin, a bonus awaited us: shiny, white, crisp tapioca.

Boiled in smaller or larger pieces, this savory root vegetable could either stand alone or be mashed with spices and coconut, then served with mutton, fish or vegetable curry or with **crushed hot green chilies**. Serving as a very inexpensive starchy root, it **became a staple food** of the locals and sustained many families for **centuries**. One plant could provide enough food to feed a **whole family** for several meals.

These same tapioca patches would become playing fields for my young cousins and I as we walked in their shade, donning tapioca leaf necklaces and hibiscus stamen ear rings, all the while pretending to be brides, fair maidens and princesses from the fairy tales the elders told us. Back then, tapioca leaf necklaces were one of the first craft lessons a child was introduced to by mothers or other older females and was often used to distract a child when she was sad or unruly. By skillfully breaking the stem into small pieces **without tearing off the** skin and dividing it into two long strings, one could easily fashion this attractive piece of do-it-yourself jewelry. Tearing off the ends the leaf fingers to make a short circle would create a pendant where the two stem strands met. A piece of sharp dry thin twig pierced into the stem on either side held the necklace together on the neck. Hibiscus stamen stems were sticky when crushed and could be stuck on to earlobes with ease. The princess's wardrobe was now complete.

Tapioca, originally from South America, was introduced to Kerala in 1860 by the King of Travancore (southern Kerala), who reportedly was also an avid botanist. During the Second World War, there was a shortage of rice in Kerala when the Japanese occupied Burma (now called Myanmar), and tapioca was introduced as a cheap source of starch for the masses.

During my recent, yearly trips to Kerala, I was saddened and heartened at the same time when I saw the sparkle and delight in a five-year old's eyes as I sat on the steps of Ahimsa Retreat and introduced the "Tapioca Leaf Necklace" to her, her older siblings watching with curious delight. The children of Kerala are no more familiar with the tapioca necklace or the Hibiscus earrings. Most of their time is spent hypnotized in the glow of their computers or cell phones while their parents spend their leisure transfixed in front of a television set.

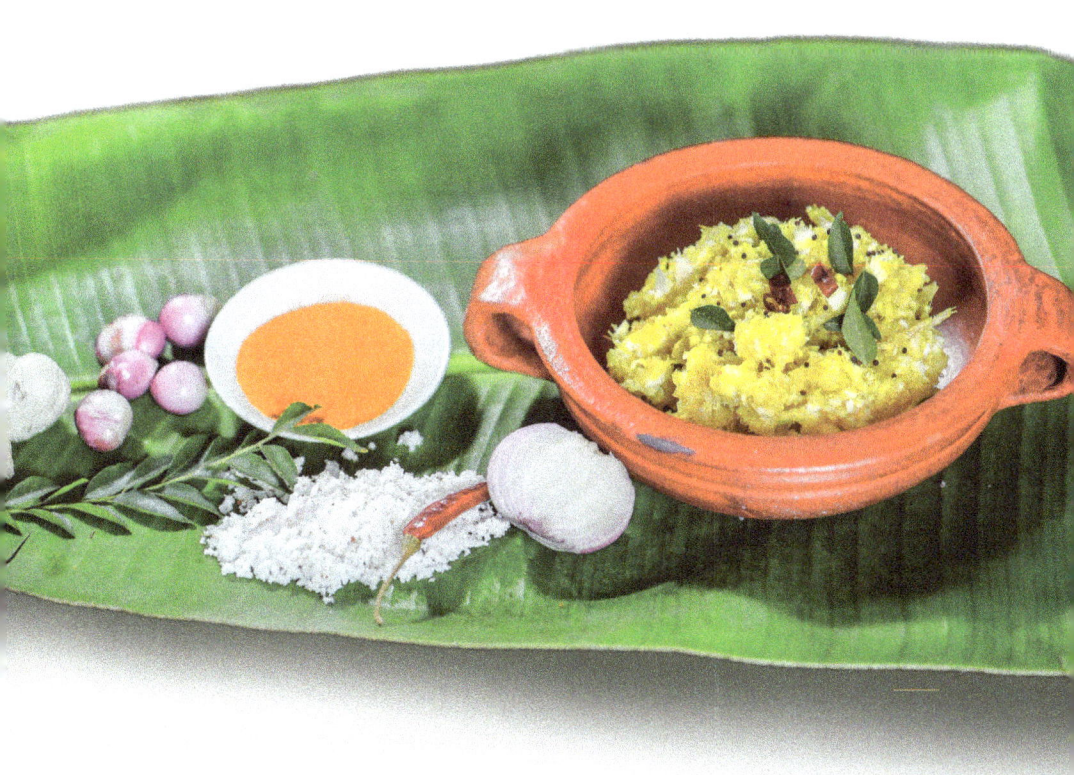

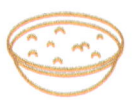

Spiced Mashed Tapioca
Kappa Veakichhade

Ingredients

- 1 Pound Tapioca Root Peeled washed and cut into 3-inch pieces
- 2-3 cloves of garlic crushed
- 1 green chili (optional, omit if cannot tolerate spicy heat)
- 1 tbsp peeled crushed ginger
- 1 cup fresh grated coconut
- 1 tbsp chopped red onion
- 10-15 fresh curry leaves
- ½ tsp turmeric
- 1 tbsp coconut oil

Process

- Boil tapioca roots in enough water to heat the contents until cooked to crushable consistency like a baked potato.
- Drain.
- Crush garlic, onion and green chili slightly in a mortar.
- Add all ingredients except coconut oil to the cooked tapioca.
- Add 1/2 cup of water and steam in medium heat for 4-5 minutes or until most of water disappears.
- Add salt to taste, and mash the tapioca and mix contents with a wooden spoon.
- While mixture is still hot, pour coconut oil over the top of the mix.

Serve hot by itself or with a curry, hot sauce or gravy of choice. Best with Keralan fish curry.

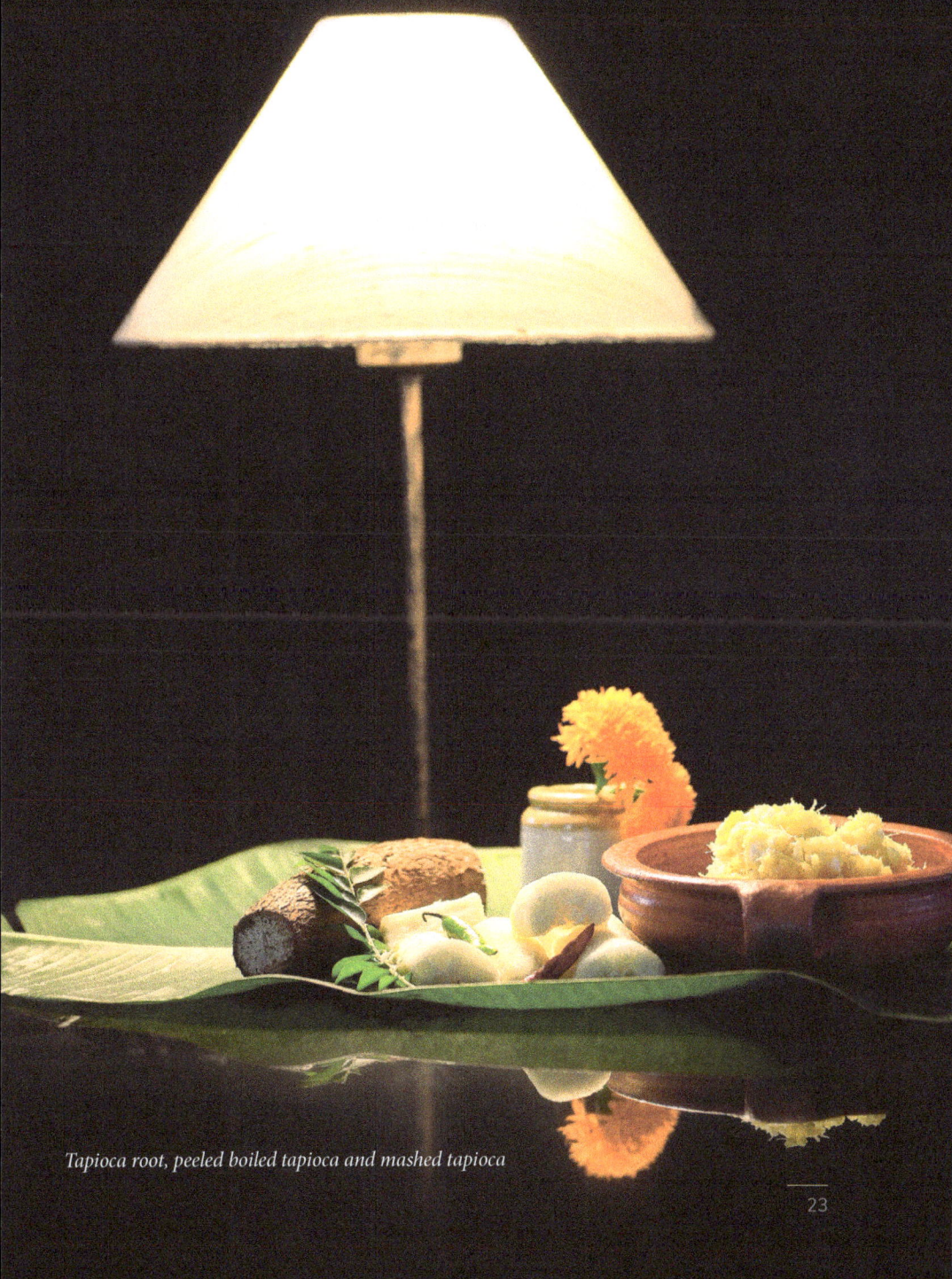
Tapioca root, peeled boiled tapioca and mashed tapioca

BANANA LEAF WRAPPED BAKED FISH ROE
(baked in ashes)
Charattil Chutta Parinjil

Summer vacations at the ancestral home took place in the Kerala backwaters, a huge eco-system that encompasses over 550 square miles of rivers, canals and paddy fields. These sites always flood between harvests and drain into lakes, deltas, lagoons and estuaries, all of which eventually empty into the Arabian Sea.

The unique ecology of this massive system sustains a complex, diverse and often precariously-balanced assortment of freshwater and marine life, one that is truly a rarity. At or below sea level, salt water from the Arabian Sea seeps into many of these waterways during the hot and dry summer months of April and May. This seasonal change makes the water brackish and encourages coastal and inward migration of many marine fish. It also creates conditions for crustaceans, such as shrimp and prawn, to flourish in the inland lakes and extensive, waterlogged paddy fields.

These marine fish often return to the sea after their brief foray along the coast and into some of these watershed landscapes. Starting in June, monsoon rains make rivers and streams of the backwaters swell, reversing the direction of flow back toward the ocean, and it is during this time that spawning season begins. Fish—especially those swollen with roe—become plentiful when this happens. That's the time of year that Grandma's hearth produced the most precious and delectable, ancient recipe: **Charattil chutta prinjil,** fish roe cooked in hot ashes.

On those evenings when the sun disappeared and the sky sparkled with swirls of stars of the Milky Way, other noises were drowned out as the chirping of the crickets got louder. The candles were lit in preparation for the recital of the rosary and other evening prayers. The altar consisted of a wooden chest in the middle of the floor of the verandah.

> *Etched into my memory of those days are images of the wooden panel of the verandah where on one side hung a picture of the Holy Family (Mary and Joseph with the infant Jesus in the middle). A framed print of John F. Kennedy took pride of place on the other side of the panel. Catholic families in Kerala were very proud of our first Catholic-American president. All would be right with the world.*

By this point in the day, my grandfather's most important task would have already been completed. At dusk, he would set out with his fishing net and copper pot. With one sweeping, circular throw, the net would land in the river, then slowly drop into the water, weighed down by a border of metallic beads. Schools of roe-filled **choora** and other freshwater fish were pulled up into the net as he skillfully navigated it back to the bank. The pot, now full to overflowing with jumping and wiggling fish, was handed over to Grandma and her assistants at the kitchen's side door.

This only took place on those days when the water-borne "market" was not active. At those times, Grandpa would skip the fishing routine as roe-filled sardines or mackerel had already been delivered by fisherman who had arrived in mini-canoes earlier in the day.

On the days, however, when our catch of fish depended upon him, Grandpa would jump into the river for a quick rinse when he was done. After his bathing ritual, he would then proceed to occupy his easy chair on the other side of the verandah, our signal that the time for prayer had arrived. From this point on and until the completion of worship, solemnity ruled, and for the next ninety minutes, the murmured sounds of faithful devotion filled the air. As that time drew to a close, however, our contemplative cadence began to accelerate, as the room filled with the distinct and magnetic aroma of the hot rice and fish curry that had begun to waft our way. An alluring meal was at hand.

As we sat cross-legged on floor-height, flat wooden seats, a freshly-washed banana leaf was placed in front of each of us, and one of the aunts would serve a steaming mound of rice on it, over which another would pour a ladle of fish curry. A beautiful golden-orange color, the curry sauce was made from chili peppers, ginger, turmeric and other spices and then blended into a waiting bowl of stone-ground coconut cream.

This fabulous fare would have been enough to satisfy us without additional touches, but during these abundant and joyful days, Grandma was able to surprise us all the more with an extra special treat. Bending over with a rapt sense of purpose, Grandma dug through the hot ashes of the wooden stove and fished out charred, banana leaf-wrapped pockets, covered in hot ash. As we waited with baited breath, as each of us slowly opened them, ultimately revealing an invaluable treasure within: baked fish roe with grated coconut, ginger and fresh local spices: **Charattil Chutta Prinjil**.

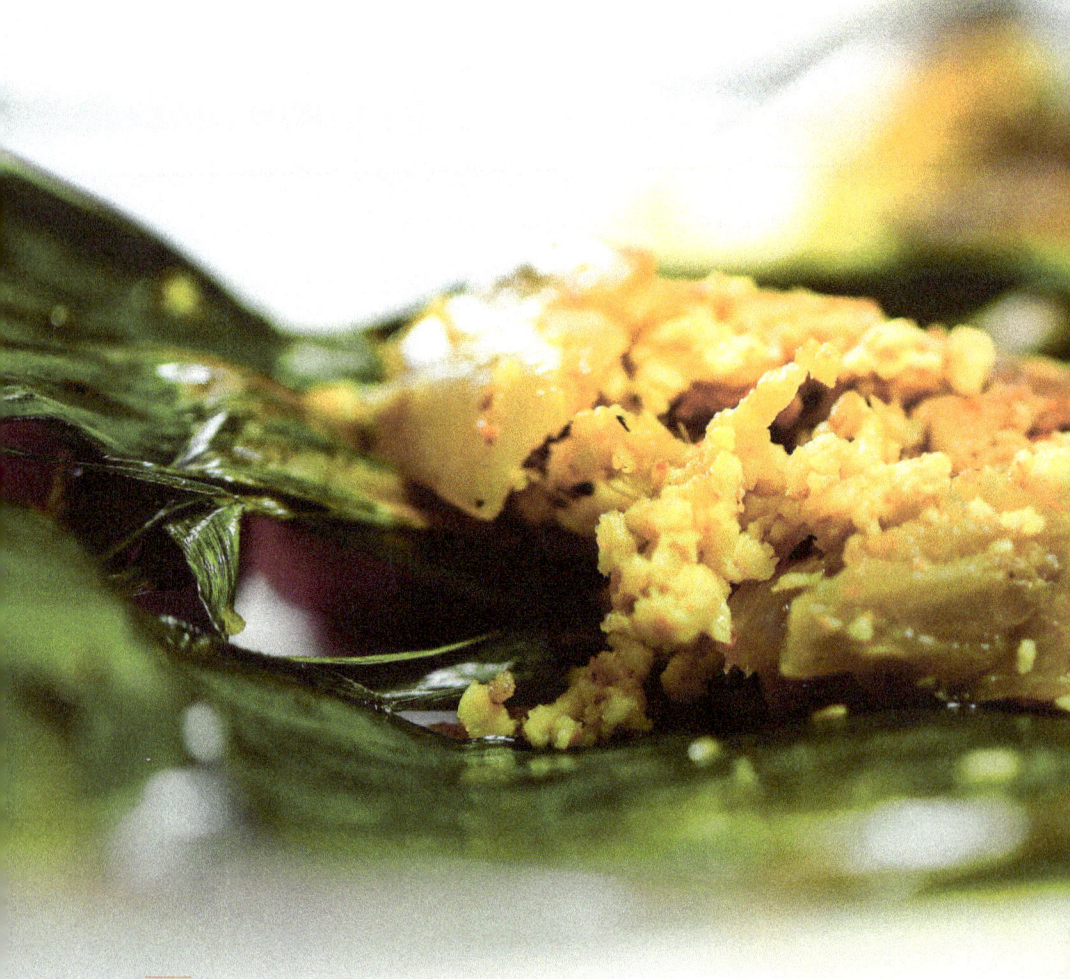

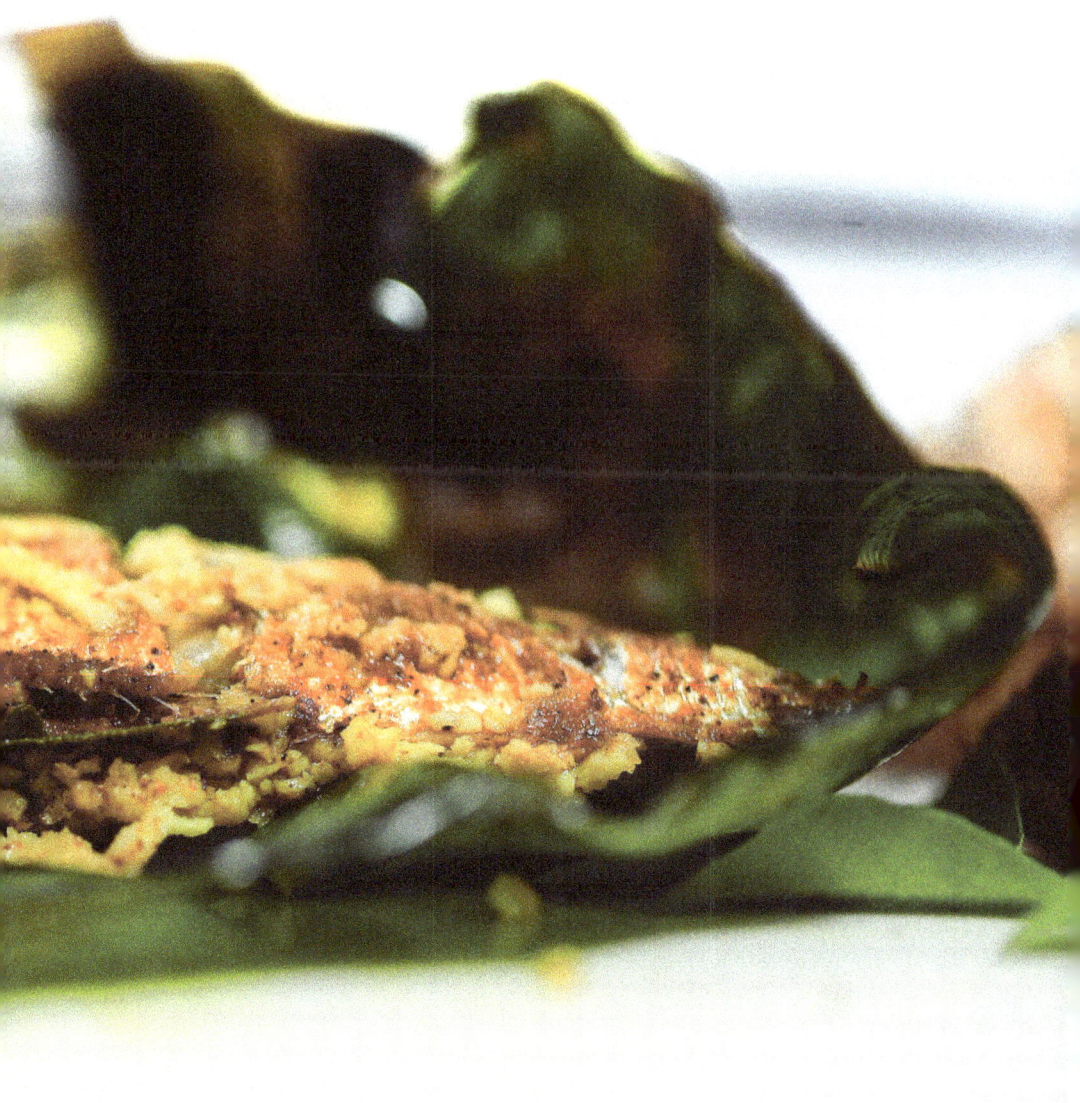

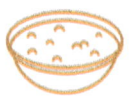

Banana Leaf Wrapped Baked Fish Roe
Modified for modern cooking

Ingredients

Fresh Banana Leaf 8x8 inch x 8

Toothpicks

1 pound raw fish roe (if not available any fish can be substituted)

1 cup fresh or frozen grated coconut

½ medium sized red onion chopped

2 tbsp grated ginger

2 green chilies chopped (optional)

1 tbsp curry leaves (2 tbsp of cilantro can be substituted if curry leaves not available)

1 tsp turmeric

½ tsp paprika

½ to 1 tsp salt to taste.

1 tsp freshly ground black pepper

1 lemon, cut into thin slices (Kerala Tamarind, **Kudampuli,** not easily available, was used in the original recipe)

Process

- Cut or carefully break the fish roe into small nuggets and gently mix all ingredients except lemon together with a fork
- Place 2-3 tbsp of of the above mixture on banana leaf.
- Place one small slice of lemon in each wrap.
- Wrap into a square packet and pin with a toothpick.
- If wooden stove or BBQ ash available, can bury in the hot ashes for 5-8 min.

Other options

Place the wraps in a bamboo steamer or other steamer and steam for 8-10 min. Or bake in oven 375 F for 10-15 min.

Serve with hot rice or on top of toast.

Fish roe substituted with fresh Sardine for this Recipe

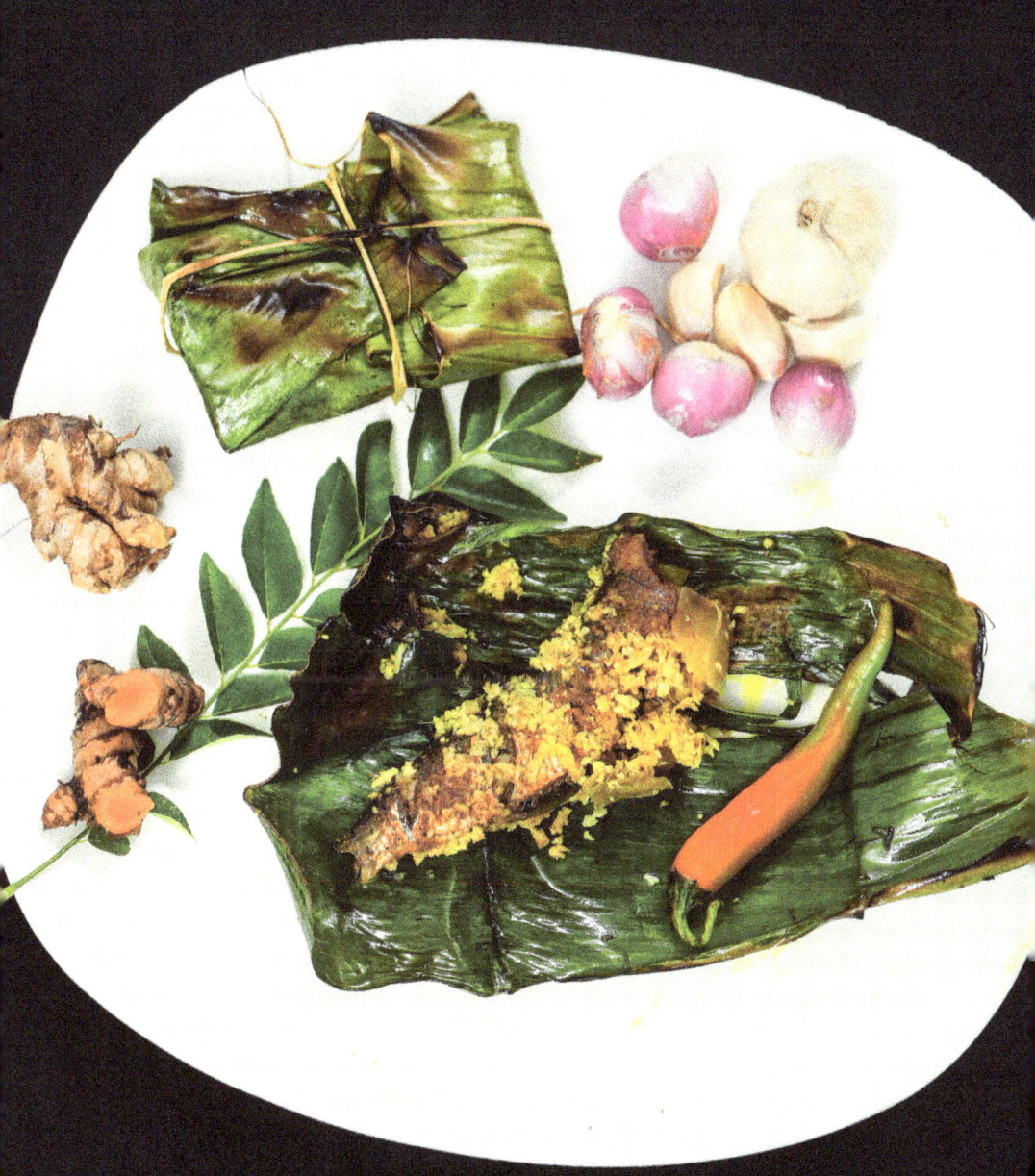

Banana leaf wrapped baked sardine

GRANDMA'S SHRIMP CURRY & STEAMED SHRIMP
Konju Curry & Konju Pattichhade

Flanked by the Arabian Sea, Indian Ocean and the Bay of Bengal and capped by the formidable Himalayan ranges to the north, lies India, the vast, triangular body of land. Its mountainous, upper region forms a barrier, enabling warm, equatorial winds to bathe its more southerly provinces with consistent, year-round balminess.

When the spring equinox is reached and then passes, the relentless sun begins its inexorable, northward shift, and winds from the south drift over the entirety of this colossal land mass, driven by the low pressure created in the great northern plains. This results in an intense, dry heat as the tall Himalayan ranges obstruct the cooler polar winds from the north. These same natural forces bring moisture-laden winds to the south, heralding the famous monsoons. The natives of Kerala greet these drenching proceedings in June or July once the very humid, hot summer months of April and May have departed. One can watch as the clouds gather and intense lightning and thunder give way to sheets of blinding, savage rain, the deluge causing streams to swell with meters of flooding in minutes.

The end of the monsoon season, in September, announces the peak spawning season, when fish are found in abundance. Shellfish—including small shrimp and giant Grandpa Shrimp (as they were called locally), many up to a foot in length, and heavily whiskered—were plentiful during my childhood years in the 1960s and early 1970s. During this time in my life, rice was grown on the low-lying paddy fields of the Kerala backwaters only every other year. As a result, much of time, the paddy fields were intentionally flooded between plantings and served as an excellent breeding ground for aquatic species, including native shellfish, which typically spawned only in the nearby freshwater, Vembanad lake, and into which emptied many local rivers and streams before making their way out to the ocean.

In those days, the conditions in the flooded paddy fields allowed the spawning of various types of shrimp much closer to home. During these times, shrimp showed up in ample quantities, enriching the meals of landlords and laborers alike. Grandpa appeared then, flush with buckets of these marvelous crustaceans, the whiskers of a few "grandpa" shrimp sticking out above the rim of the bucket, showing off his seasonal bonus with pride.

There was no electricity or refrigeration back then, so Grandma would boil the shrimp with turmeric, green chilies, curry leaves, and a special Kerala tamarind, known as **kudampuli**, in large clay **Urilis**. The shrimp were then well preserved, and could be taken out in small quantities for use in various dishes that Grandma would prepare in the ensuing weeks.

Hot summer afternoons—the time when children would spend vacation at the ancestral home—were a time when youthful mischief abounded. As Grandma faded into her afternoon slumber the more brazen among us slipped into her room, hoping to get in and out with a sampling of the surreptitiously placed, shrimp-laden *Urli*, which had been slyly covered in banana leaves and hidden under her bed.

My cousin Raju had mastered this craft. Slender of foot and skilled of hand, he would crawl under Grandma's bed, exceedingly careful to be mindful so as not to upset her repose, and, using bits of banana leaf as a napkin, deftly grasp a fistful of the contents of the **Urli**. Once an appropriate quantity of stolen delights was acquired, we children would run off to the far end of the property, bordered by the flooded paddy fields. We had an epic, late-day picnic of shrimp on banana leaves, licking our fingertips and savoring the very last bit of remaining flavor. This continued for many days, whenever possible, until the **Urli** was left pathetically empty, with only the scratchy remains of mostly turmeric-stained, curry leaves and green chili, testifying to its former glory. All was well, until Grandma, in preparation for her next succulent shrimp dish, pulled out the miserably barren **Urli** from under the bed.

At these times, when we children were markedly afraid that our crime would be noticed, we avoided coming anywhere near the house until late in the evening, hoping that Grandma would be too busy preparing dinner to dole out any punishment. Not one to be readily mollified, Grandma stood at the ready with her slender bamboo stick (**chooravadi**), which she kept in an undisclosed place, awaiting the day when one of us would require discipline. She chased us throughout the house, then into the yard, stick firmly in hand, until she finally gave up in exhaustion, as the younger women of the house laughed at the spectacle. Sometimes one among them would join in, attempting to assist Grandma in capturing the culprits, who most often managed to escape to the safety of the deep and expansive backyard.

For the next few days shrimp disappeared from our plates and was replaced by our least favorite vegetable dishes, such as stir-fried Banana Flowers (Coombu) or spinach and some times mere coconut chutney and rice. That was, of course, until the next batch of **Urli** was ready.

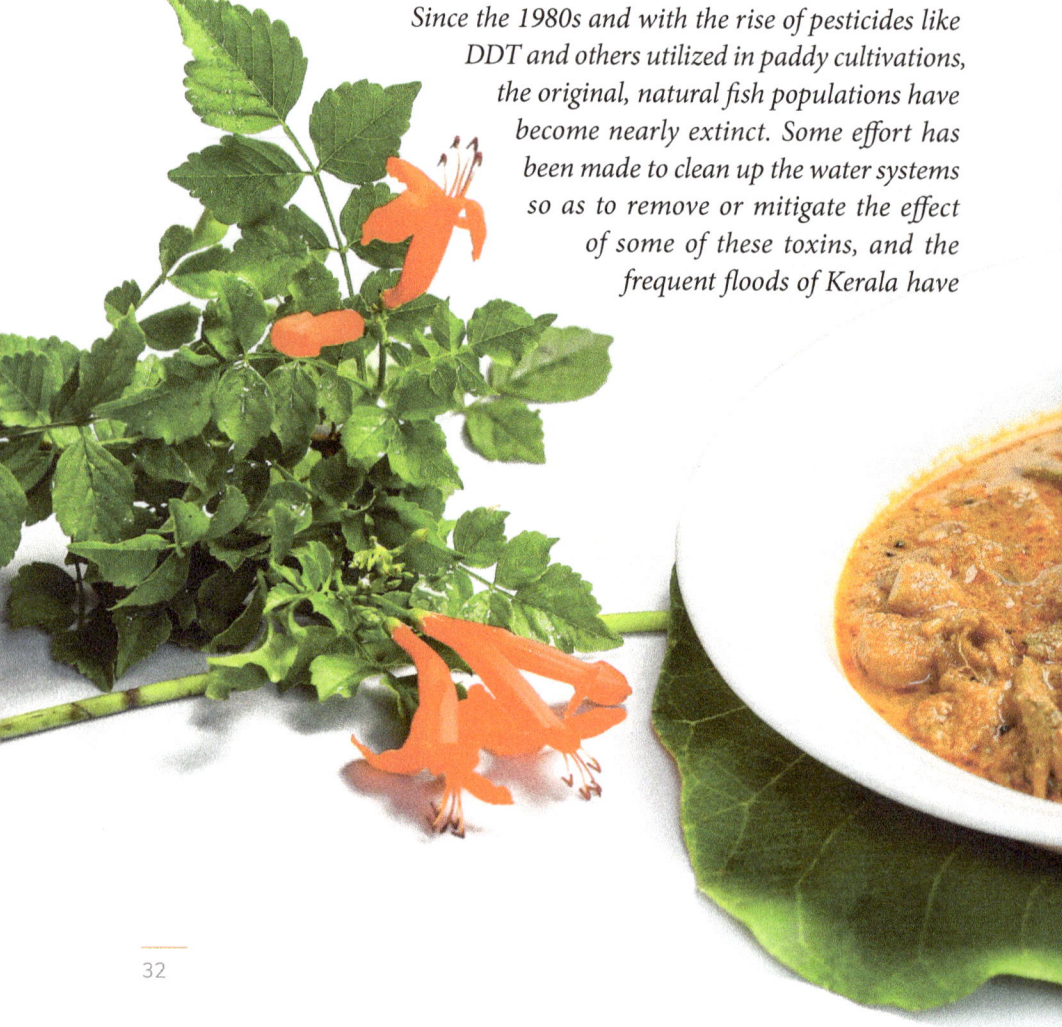

Since the 1980s and with the rise of pesticides like DDT and others utilized in paddy cultivations, the original, natural fish populations have become nearly extinct. Some effort has been made to clean up the water systems so as to remove or mitigate the effect of some of these toxins, and the frequent floods of Kerala have

generally benefited this endeavor. To counteract the devastation wrought on the native fish population, some species are now artificially generated and maintained by government hatcheries.

Grandma's fish dishes, and all of the wonderful and sundry experiences surrounding them, beacon from a different time and place, and I find myself, as I wend my way toward our modern day "Organic Grocery Stores," trying, but often failing, to recreate the tastes and smells of that bygone era. Brutal and uncompromising optimism leads me to believe though that, against all odds, and at some grassroots level, we will slowly but surely retrace our steps. I hope we will get off our comfortable chairs and away from our iPhones and our Macs, distracted as we are by FaceTime and Instagram to pay attention. I pray, in their place, that we engage in Realtime with Real People so that our children and our children's children will experience the simple joys that keep us grounded and content during our brief sojourn on this Earth.

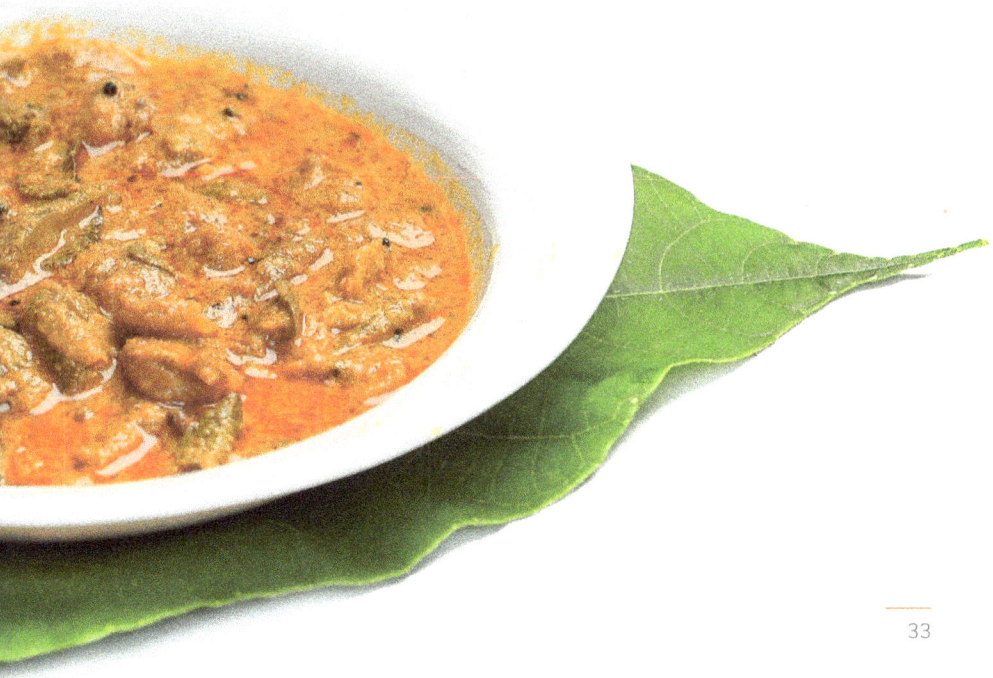

Grandma's Shrimp Curry
Konju Curry

Ingredients

1 pound medium sized shrimp.

1 can organic coconut milk 8 oz. (*if fresh or frozen grated coconut available 1 cup grated coconut or coconut pieces blended finely in blender with water is the best*)

½ inch cube fresh ginger, crushed or grated

2 cloves of garlic crushed

½ medium sized red onion finely diced

½ cup tomatoes finely diced

1 - stem or 15-20 curry leaves (*if not available, substitute cilantro as garnish*)

1-2 tbsp cooking oil of choice (coconut oil is the best)

1 tsp mustard seeds

1 tbsp coarsely crushed fennel seed

1 dried red chili broken in half

1 tsp turmeric

1 tsp paprika powder

½ tsp to 1 tsp chili pepper (*if spice not tolerated substitute with few dashes of black pepper*)

1 tbsp coriander powder

Salt to taste

Process

- Wash shrimp with running cold water for 3-4 min and keep drained in a colander.
- If using grated coconut, blend coconut, ginger, garlic and tomatoes to a fine paste in a blender and put aside. If using coconut milk, use 1/4 cup of coconut milk and blend the same ingredients and put aside.
- Heat oil in a deep frying pan or wok.
- Place mustard and dried red chili in hot oil keep covered loosely with gap or mesh lid until mustard pops.
- Add washed dried curry leaves.
- Add remaining onions and stir until brown.
- Add coriander powder and stir constantly for 1 minute, then lower heat to minimum.
- Add paprika and turmeric to the oil stirring constantly for 1-3 minutes.

- Add paste from the blender and cook stirring constantly in medium heat for 3-5 min until mixture exudes a roasted smell.
- Add shrimp and stir on low-med heat for 2-3 minutes.
- Add remaining coconut milk from the can (*or water, 1-2 cups of water if grated coconut was used instead of canned coconut milk*).
- Add more water if needed until shrimp are barely immersed in the sauce.
- Add salt to taste.
- Heat uncovered on medium heat until mixture boils.
- Lower heat and cover and cook on low heat for 5-8 min (*do not overcook; check shrimp for consistency, and turn off heat when shrimp are soft but not mushy. Overcooking will make shrimp rubbery and less tasty*).
- Add crushed fennel.
- Add more salt to desired taste if needed.
- *Garnish with coriander leaves if curry leaves not available.*

Serve hot with rice.

Sardines, mackerel, clams, mussels and other salt water fish can also be cooked using the same recipes.

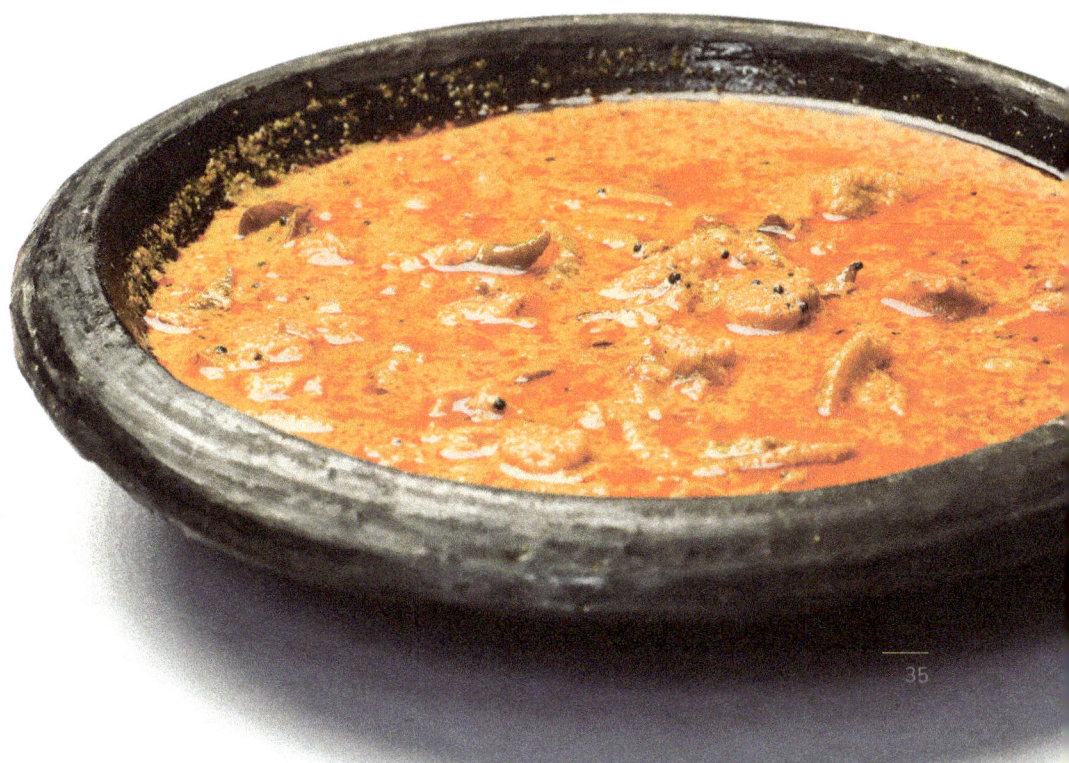

Grandma's Steamed Shrimp
Konju Pattichade

Ingredients

1 pound cleaned peeled and deveined shrimp (may substitute with fresh sardines—whole, cleaned, and degutted—or mackerel fillet, sliced into pieces 1-2 inch

½ medium sized red onion chopped

2 tbsp grated ginger

2 green chilies chopped (optional if cannot tolerate spice), or leave whole partially sliced lengthwise

1 tbsp curry leaves (2 tbsp of cilantro can be substituted if curry leaves not available)

½ cup grated coconut (available frozen in Indian grocery stores)

1 tsp turmeric

1 tsp freshly ground black pepper

¼ tsp Paprika (optional)

3-4 dashes of Asafetida if available (optional)

1 lemon thinly sliced circles or 2-3 quarter-sized slivers of dried Kerala Tamarind (*Kudampuli*)

Salt to taste

Process

- If using Kerala Tamarind, wash and soak Tamarind in ½ cup of hot water. Add ¼ tsp salt and keep aside.

- Mix all above ingredients (except lemon or Tamarind, mentioned above) gently with hand in a pan.

- Pour Tamarind, if used, into the mixture. If using lemon instead of Tamarind, add ½ cup of water to mixture and spread lemon pieces over the top.

- Cook covered over high heat until boiling, which takes 3-5 minutes and then turn heat to low.

- Cook for 8-10 min covered on low heat. Check periodically and add 2-3 tbsp of water to keep mixture moist and prevent from burning. Remove mixture from heat and keep covered until ready to serve.

This dish gets better the next day and can be served for 2-3 days. Best served with rice.

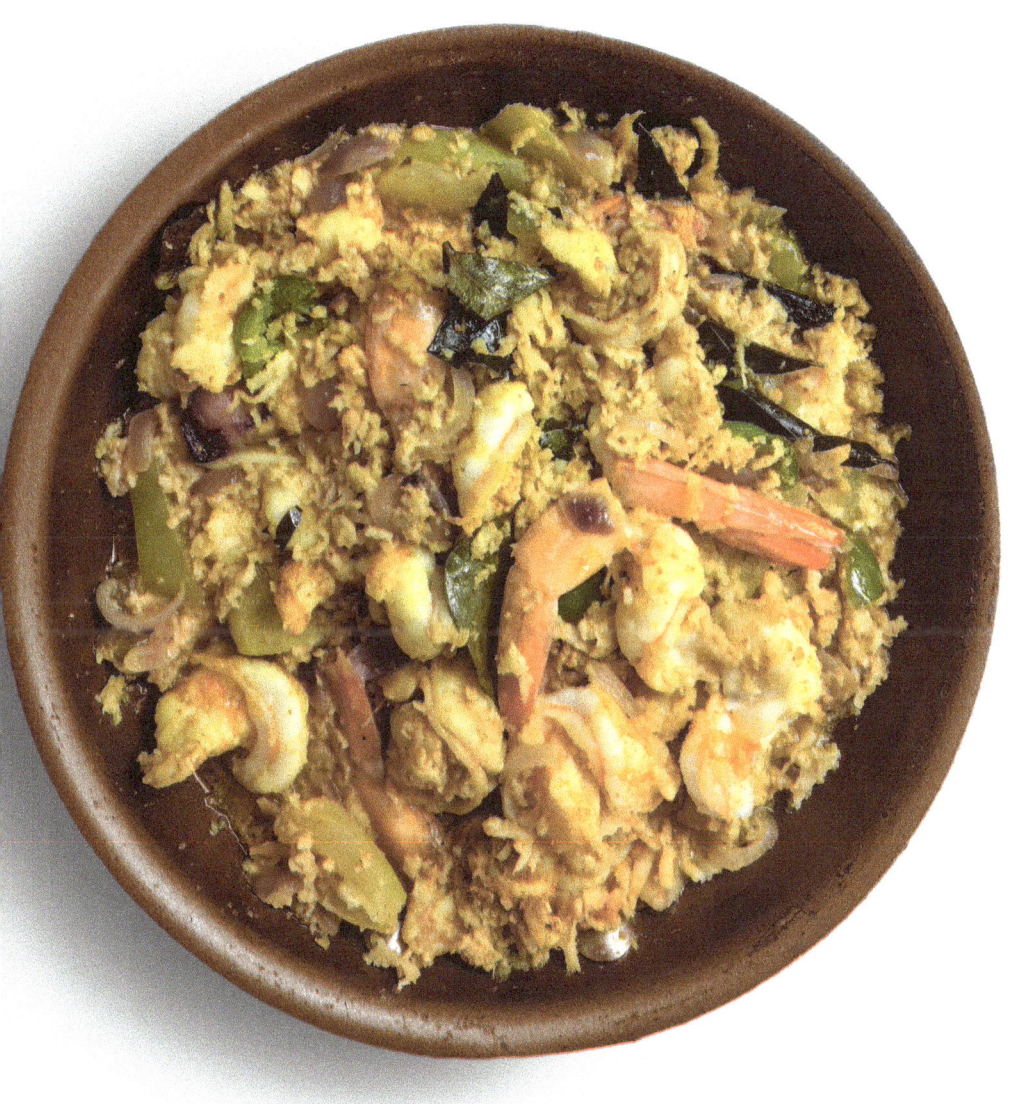

CREPES ROASTED IN BANANA LEAF
Elel Parattiya Appam

At our home in the backwaters of Kerala, the family and neighbors would affectionately refer to me as *"Elel Parattiya Appam."* This was because it was well known that, even at a very young age, I followed my grandmother Theresa around, begging her to make me these irresistible crepes of the same name.

What made this wonderful dish inescapably compelling? It may have been the crispy, chewy texture offered with each bite. Perhaps it was the rich, nutty, sweet and earthy aroma that crept into my brain, proclaiming and giving rise to something entirely wholesome and satisfying. Or maybe it was the simple fact that no one could make it quite like Grandma, for she was the only one who could judge the heat of the skillet accurately, and she was the only one who knew how to apply the perfect amount of pressure with her sturdy, wrinkled fingers so that the dough took to the skillet like a second skin, metamorphosing into a heavenly manna.

It was only Grandma who knew when to turn the crepe over, just in time to allow it to cook perfectly, its flavor and texture impeccable from years of practice. When made in traditional fashion, the dough was pressed over a banana leaf, but my personal preference was to have this dough cooked directly on the skillet, baked to perfection by the direct conduction of heat via its wrought iron surface. The crepes, which are called Ada, when made this way seemed to come out chewier and crispier.

When I was very young and up until the age of nine, I was the only grandchild that came from a faraway place to spend the summers in Kerala. The other cousins arrived from nearby villages and towns, and I was therefore considered somewhat of a celebrity. This afforded me special privileges, not the least of which was being served **Ada** on demand. This was no small triumph as making the dough for it was quite laborious and time consuming.

To get ready for summer vacation visitors, the aunts in the house would begin the preparations: fresh, raw mango, ginger, lemon, and bitter gourd pickles would be crafted and placed in classic oval, beige and brown porcelain jars well in advance. Gooseberries, pickled in honey or molasses, jackfruit halwa, and other sweetmeats would also be readied or bought from the Changanacherry market, then stocked in the corner pantry of Grandma's bedroom. The paddy would also be milled and pounded into powder then roasted and stored for dishes like **Ada**.

I became deeply attached to this dish the very first time I tasted it, and it became the symbol by which I could gauge Grandma's affection. If she gave me the best of the batch, if she put extra coconut in mine, or if she was willing to go out of her way and make one special batch just for me when others had to settle for something ordinary, I knew that I occupied a unique and dear place in Grandma's heart. When I was indulged, I luxuriated in that feeling, and when I was not, I would pout, cry and demonstrate true hurt, thereby earning the namesake nickname, **Elel Parattiya Appum!**

To this day, I beam with joy when, upon returning to my own home in Kerala, our cook Saraswati surprises me with a piping hot **Ada,** sprinkled with brown sugar with evening tea. At that moment, and especially when the chaos of daily life threatens to overtake me, this precious offering helps me escape into the innocence and joy of childhood as I crunch, munch and inhale its sweet, soothing fragrance and bathe in a sea of life-affirming memories and experiences.

Elel Parattiya Appam

Best served with evening Kerala Coffee | Makes 4 Crepes

Ingredients

Fresh banana leaf, 8x8 inch square (optional, can make the crepe directly on the skillet too)

2 cups coarsely ground parboiled rice (can also be substituted with cream of wheat)

¾ cup fresh grated coconut

½ tsp cumin seed

½ tsp salt

1-2 tbsp brown sugar (optional)

Hot water

Process

- Roast ground rice powder (or cream of wheat) in an iron skillet or wok for 3-5 minute, stirring constantly with spatula until you can smell roasted grain aroma. Keep aside until the powder has cooled down.
- Mix ingredients (add brown sugar if you want to make sweet Ada) with small amounts of water to make a dough like consistency. Do not knead too much; leave air pockets.
- Heat a large, cast iron skillet. Place banana leaf on skillet and lower heat.
- Pat and flatten a 2-inch ball of above dough to a thin layer with finger tips onto the banana leaf until most of the leaf is covered except 1/2 inch along the edges. Alternatively, dough can be applied directly to the skillet as explained above to make **Ada** and skip the immediate next step.
- Fold the leaf with dough in half and flatten over the leaf gently with a wooden spoon or spatula.
- Raise heat slightly; cook on one side for 2-3 min pressing down gently.
- Flip over and do the same until the crepe seems crisp and the aroma of roasted grain and banana leaf fills the kitchen.

*Serve for breakfast or evening snack with **Chai** or Kerala black coffee.*

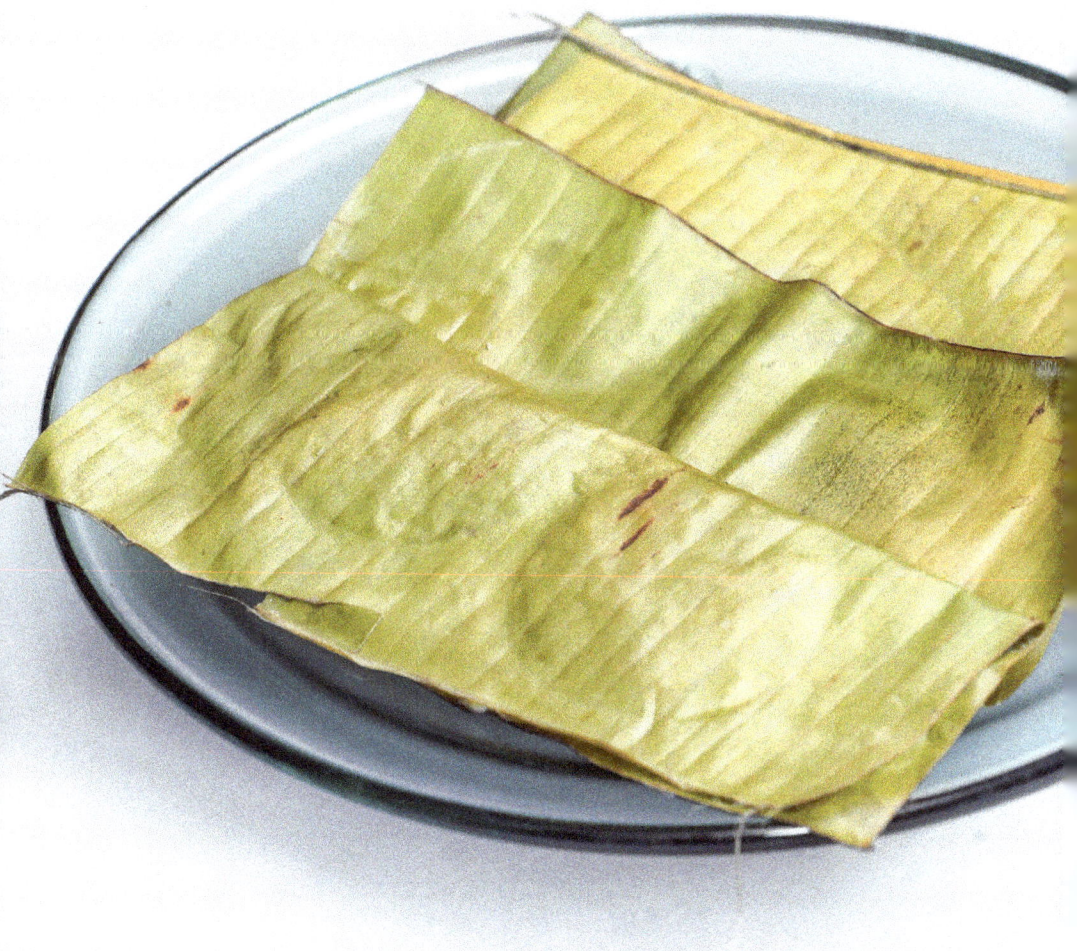

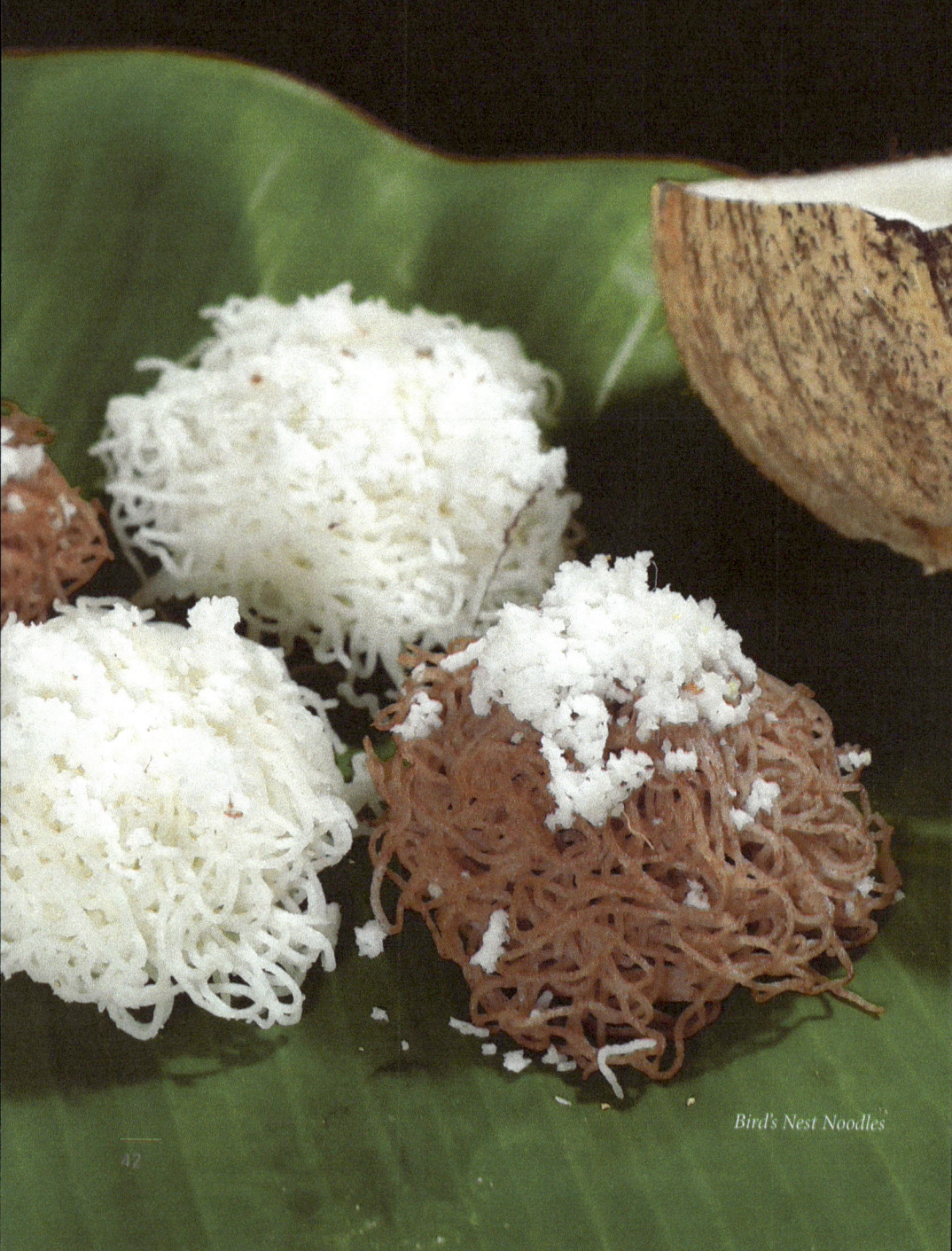

Bird's Nest Noodles

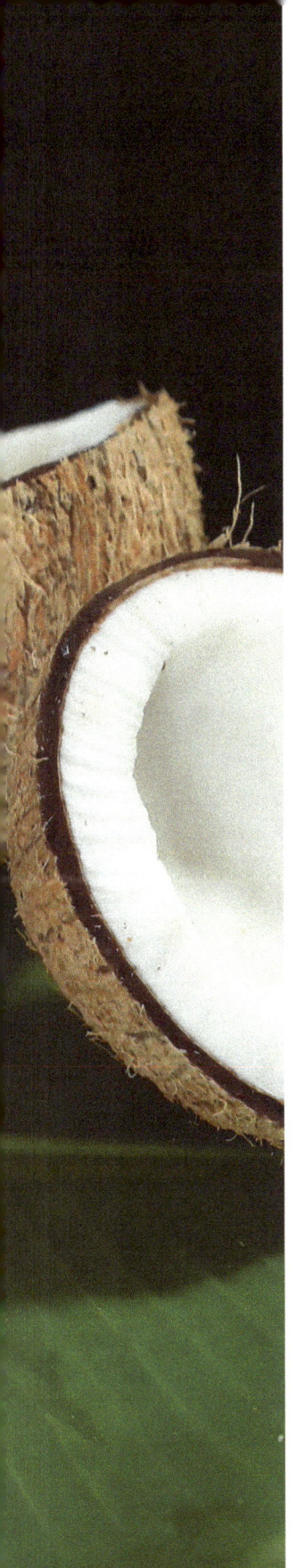

BREAKFAST

MIRIAM AND MALI'S CASHEW AND RAISIN OATMEAL

During the seventeen years I spent growing up in India, I never ate oatmeal. Later, in America, I realized that the gruel served to the orphans featured in old black and white renditions of Charles Dickens' *Oliver Twist* was perhaps one and the same. Oatmeal had a most unappealing appearance in those grainy images, and I never made its acquaintance.

All this changed, years later, when **Aunt Miriam**, my mother's elder sister, and **Amma Mali,** my mother-in-law, both then in their mid-fifties, arrived from Kerala and Mumbai to care for my newborn son in America while I completed my medical residency, working twenty to thirty hour shifts.

Aunt Miriam, hailing as she did from a frugal, Keralan Catholic family, where gluttony was considered a mortal sin, was an exceptionally finicky eater. She ingested extremely small portions, and only ate food that agreed with her taste buds. This suited both her conscience and her constitution. She was a tall, thin woman, measuring almost six feet tall, with a flawless, radiant, olive complexion and shiny locks of curly black hair. People said that she was one of the most beautiful women in the village. She was the prettiest of my mother's three sisters. Her relationship with food may have explained her long healthy life. The most I ever heard her complain about was a pain in her left shoulder. X-rays taken in America later revealed an old undiagnosed fracture that healed spontaneously. As far as she could recall, it most likely happened when she was a young bride. She suffered a fall while attempting to restrain a cow chasing its calf.

Then there was **Amma Mali**, who also arrived to help with my son. She planned to arrive when Aunt Miriam left, and so they alternated, living with us every other year for several years. Aunt Miriam was introduced to oatmeal at a relative's house in America. She imagined that it would be agreeable to her picky palate. She decided that adding a few cumin seeds to the oatmeal would turn it into a more desirable dish.

Mali, in stark contrast to Aunt Miriam, was the regal child of a Konkani Brahmin family. This priestly caste firmly believed that food, cooking and eating were not to be taken lightly. Portions that were bigger, richer, savory, and more elaborate, were considered of the greatest worth and importance when it came to their rightful place at the table.

Mali was very short and plump. She was one of the happiest women I have ever known. Like Aunt Miriam, she too had an immaculate brown complexion, a perfectly sculpted, royal nose, and large, round sparkling eyes. Most of her activity revolved around planning and preparing rich, tasty meals. She would be considered obese by modern standards. Now, she takes medicine for a little high blood pressure and elevated cholesterol. Other than that, she has been blessed to have avoided any serious illness.

On one particularly ordinary day, Aunt Miriam offered Mali a bowl of her cumin-spiced oatmeal. She consumed it in its entirety, and thought it tasted good enough, but felt that it needed her Brahmin touches in order to turn it into a truly compelling dish. Mali added milk, cashews, raisins and ghee. Voila! A bold and compelling recipe was born, and a once humble gruel was transformed into a meal that radiated divinity.

Many years later, Amma Mali's heavenly porridge remains a favorite dish among Ahimsa Kitchen patrons, who travel from many parts of the world, including America, Britain, Japan and even India to attend Yoga and Ayurvedic retreats at Ahimsa Retreats in Kerala.

After over three decades as a Western- trained physician practicing allopathic medicine, these life experiences challenge my notion of what we consider good nutrition. Here are two individuals whose notion of food, flavor, satisfaction and spiritual and ethical connotations of food were shaped by their social and religious backgrounds and are worlds apart. Yet, they both lived long and healthy lives. The common factor is that both took the food they consumed seriously, taking care to make preparations that suited their palates as well as their philosophy of life. I could imagine Aunt Miriam falling sick trying the consume Amma Mali's oatmeal, and Mali being completely dissatisfied and unfulfilled with only Miriam's options taking away some of the quality of her life.

Modern day interpretations distort Miriam and Mali's philosophies and practices as two extremes, stripping food and cooking from its social and spiritual connotations. In the contemporary psyche, food is transformed into "calorie counts," BMIs, and cholesterol, as well as other analytical tests on a lab report. The goal is to treat the numbers and measurable indices like weight that can be catalogued and statistically analyzed. The most important factor, the quality of life, is completely neglected, and the meaning and purpose of the food is ignored.

As a result, we have, on one end of the spectrum, individuals obsessed with weight, calories and appearances, yet unhappy and sick in perfectly sculpted bodies, afraid to touch food without counting the calories. On the other end, we have individuals who consume large quantities of commercially prepared food lacking in history and context, designed only to satisfy their palate temporarily and sending them into a hyperglycemic stupor, drowning their fears, anxieties and dissatisfaction.

We could benefit from searching out and connecting with our own inner Miriam and Mali, because food is not only fuel for the body, it is also sustenance for the soul.

Miriam's Version
Low Calorie

Ingredients

- 1 cup oats (not instant)
- 1 ½ cups of water
- ¼ tsp cumin seeds
- 1 tbsp raisins (green raisins from organic stores best)
- Salt to taste
- ½ banana (optional)
- Organic brown sugar (optional) or honey.

Process

- Mix all ingredients except salt and banana and cook on high heat until mixture begins to boil.
- Lower heat and cook while stirring gently for 3-5 minutes, until cooked.
- Add more water if needed based on preferred consistency.
- Add salt to taste, and garnish with sliced banana. Serve hot.

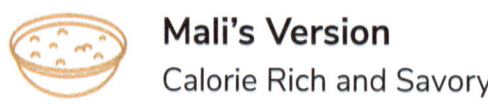

Mali's Version
Calorie Rich and Savory

Ingredients

1 cup oatmeal (not instant)

1 & ½ cups of water

¼ tsp cumin seeds

1 tbsp raisins (green raisins from organic stores are best)

10-15 cashews, halved or broken into rough pieces

1 tbsp ghee (clarified butter) or organic butter

¾ cup of milk of choice

Salt to taste

Organic brown sugar (optional) or honey

Process

- Heat ghee in a small saucepan in low-med heat.
- Add raisins and cashews and lower heat.
- Roast cashews and raisins in low heat stirring until the cashews turn lightly golden brown and the aroma of roasting cashews and ghee fill the air.
- Keep aside until oatmeal cooked.
- In a separate dish mix remaining ingredients (except salt, brown sugar or honey) and cook on high heat until begins to boil.
- Add milk.
- Lower heat and cook while stirring gently for 3-5 min.
- Add more water if needed based on preferred consistency.
- Cook on low heat stirring constantly until desired consistency.
- Add salt to taste. Mix well.
- Pour the ghee with cashews and raisins over surface of the dish.
- Sprinkle 1-2 tsp brown sugar or honey over the contents (optional).

Serve hot for breakfast.

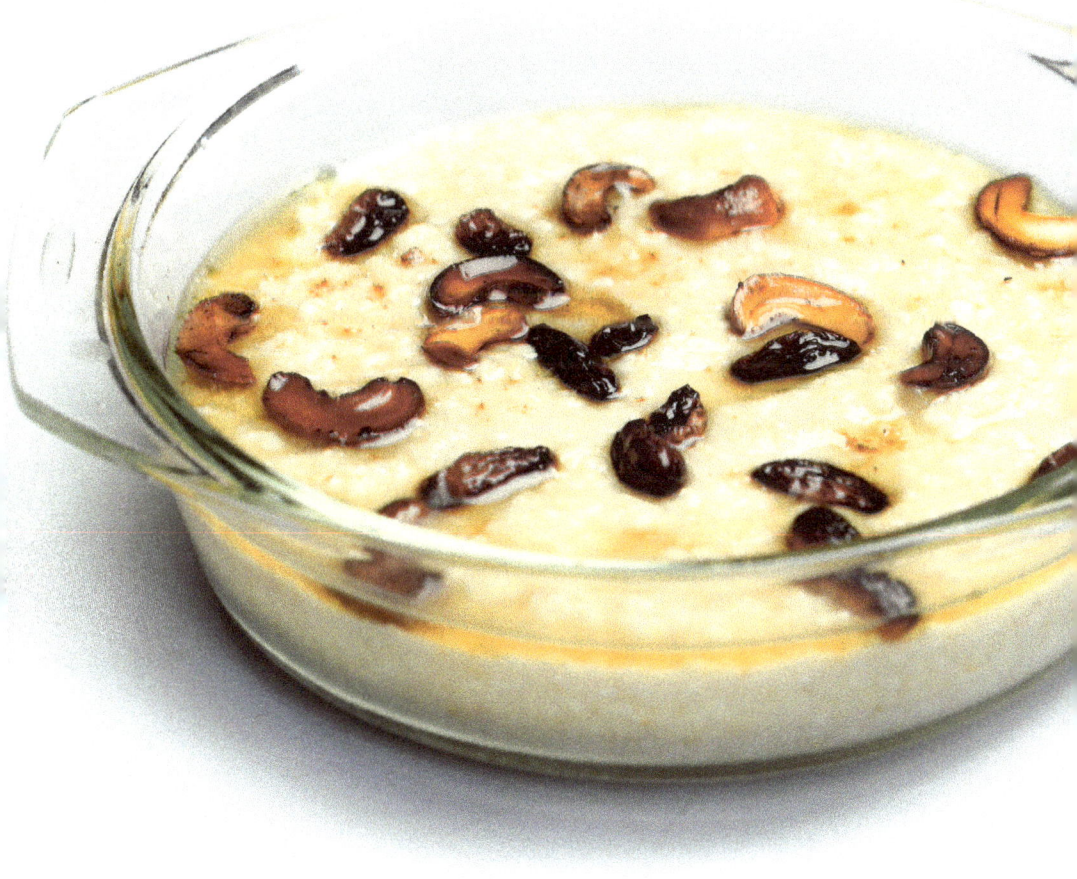

MALI AND MIRIAM'S SWEET & SAVORY VEGETABLE ROASTED CREAM OF WHEAT
Rava Upma

The history of how cream of wheat or **Rava** was introduced to South Indian Cuisine is not clear considering that wheat mainly grew in the colder climates in Northern India. I cannot remember if I first saw *Upma* as a child in my Grandma's kitchen in Kerala. I know that this dish was frequently served at our breakfast table beginning in the early 1980's when Mali and Miriam began visiting us in the USA.

Rava was a quintessential favorite of the South Indian breakfast menu especially among the Konkani and other Brahmins. Mali's special touches and laser-like attention, such as when pouring the hot water into the cream of wheat or when determining the amount of ***ghee*** she would add to the dish, were sure to produce a glistening, steaming mound of pure ambrosia. Served with either a sprinkling of sugar or a drizzle of dry coconut chutney, it was impossible to limit oneself to one serving of this fabulous concoction. Rich with peas, nuts, raisins and ***ghee***, Mali's version was luxurious and satisfying, and could lull anyone into a comatose slumber should one happen to take a second serving.

When the pantry ran out of richer ingredients, Mali would settle for a leaner yet equally succulent version, using whatever cooking oil was available or smaller quantities of butter and peas. Served regularly for breakfast and as leftovers for an evening snack, this dish never lost its fan base even after decades of living in the United States and other countries.

Miriam's version was far more measured. Her cream of wheat contained an abundance of thinly sliced carrots, beans, peas, and bits of artfully sliced vegetable leftovers. Slowly and deliberately, she gathered her ingredients, adding ghee only on special occasions. Otherwise, she would use the oil available in the kitchen. Coconut oil was her favorite. In Miriam's rendition, the cream of wheat was dry roasted, and only a small amount of water was used. It was in her gentle stirring and attention to heat that the magic of her expert craft would come to life, fragrant and nutty flavors filling our nostrils and causing our mouths to water. When tasted, Miriam's marvelous mash was not moist like Mali's, yet no less alluring. When it accompanied her brown chickpea or egg curry, it made the perfect Keralan breakfast, turning an ordinary weekday meal into a special occasion, a perfect meal to nourish the body and soul.

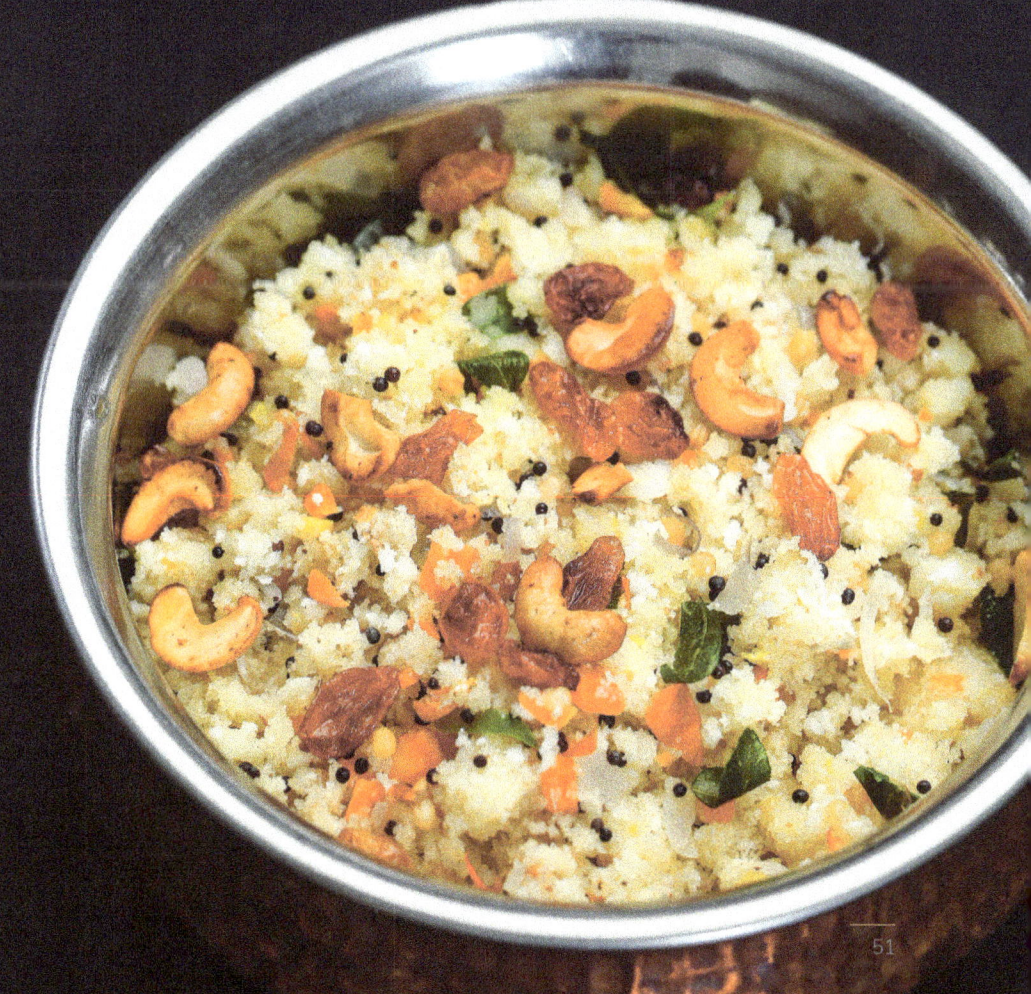

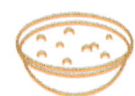

Mali's Sweet and Savory Vegetable Roasted Cream of Wheat
Rava Upma

Ingredients

2 cups cream of wheat

1-2 tbsp ghee

1 green chili whole (optional)

1/2 cup, thawed and drained frozen peas

¼ cup carrots cut into ½-inch, thin slices

1 fistful coarsely broken cashew nuts

1 tbsp black or green raisins

1 stalk fresh curry leaves (may use cilantro if curry leaves not available)

1 tsp mustard seed

1 tsp Urad Dal (optional)

2 tbsp finely chopped onion

1 tsp crushed or finely chopped ginger root

3-4 dashes Asafetida

1/2 tbsp brown cane sugar (optional)

Salt to taste

4-6 cups boiling water, keep ready for use

Process

- Heat ghee in a wok or frying pan on low to medium heat, so that the ghee does not burn.
- Roast cashews and raisins in ghee for 1-2 minutes until slightly brown; scoop out and keep in a separate dish
- Place mustard seeds and urad dal in the heated ghee. Increase heat to medium, covering lightly and leaving a gap until the mustard seeds pop. Add curry leaves and asafetida and lower heat
- Add onion, ginger, green chili, carrots and peas and 2-3 pinches of salt and cook on medium heat, stirring frequently for 3-5 minutes. Then add cream of wheat and salt to taste, stirring constantly for 2-3 minutes
- Add boiling water, stirring constantly until contents are barely immersed.
- Add the roasted nuts raisins and sugar (optional)
- Lower heat and mix thoroughly with strong wooden spoon. Add more water as needed to immerse contents slightly.

Cover with tight lid and cook on very low heat for 5-8 minutes, stir once during this last phase.

Garnish with cilantro and serve hot for breakfast or for a snack with evening tea.

Miriam's Low-calorie Savory Vegetable Roasted Cream of Wheat
Rava Upma

- Leave, cashew, raisins and sugar out from the above list. Decrease ghee by half, or use coconut or other oil, and add less water in the second to last step above.

- Cook uncovered on very low heat, stirring constantly for 3-5 minutes, then make a mound and pat it down in the middle of the frying pan. Cover with tight lid until ready to serve.

Serve with Kerala Egg Curry or Brown Chickpea Curry for a high protein, high fiber breakfast, or for any meal.

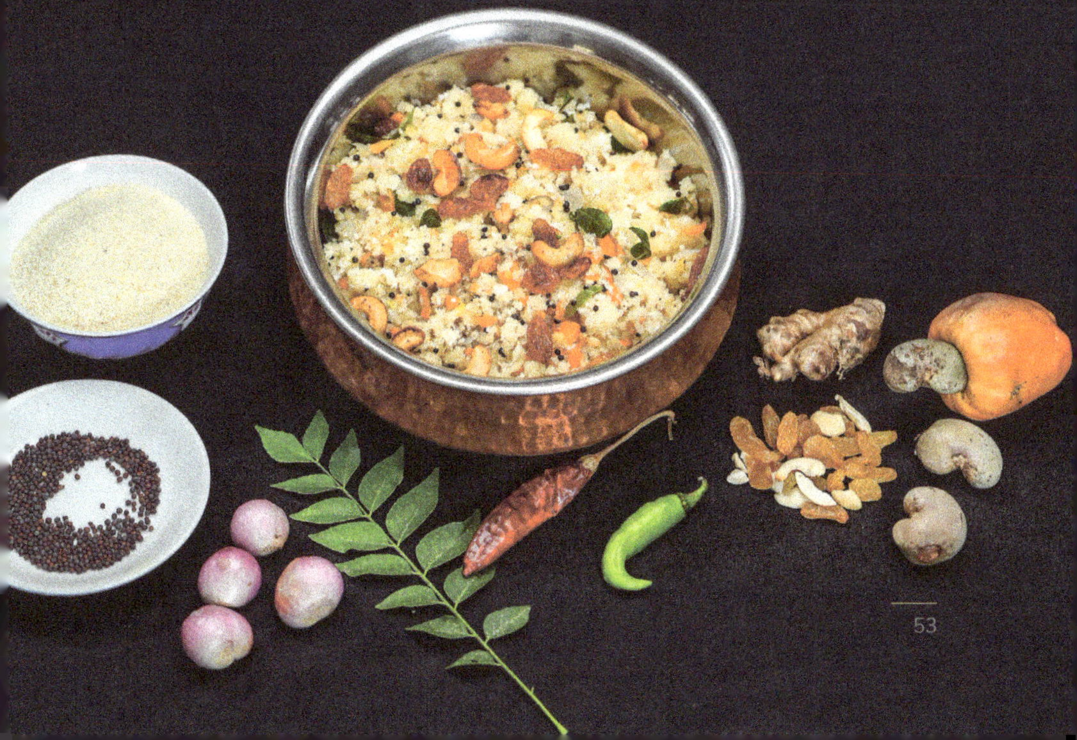

COCONUT STUFFED BIRDS NEST RICE NOODLES
Idiyappam

Served as a special Sunday dish, or as a breakfast for guests or special visitors, **Idiyappam remains** a favorite on the breakfast tables of Keralan locals and the Kerala diaspora worldwide. "*Idi*" means "pounding," while "*appam*" is actually a misnomer for this dish. It means "crepe" not "noodle."

I remember that, during childhood visits to Kerala, the preparation for **Idiyappam** began days ahead of time. Mills for grinding grains were few and far between in the village, so the women of the house would collect the requisite, parboiled paddy, still unhusked from gunny sacks in the **Ara** (the wooden room of the house where grains were stored), and then set to work, doing the milling or pounding themselves.

Afternoons in the household were quiet. Grandpa and Grandma took naps during this time; Grandpa on his easy chair on the verandah, and Grandma on her little cot in her bedroom, which doubled as a storage room, next to the kitchen. The children wandered the vast grounds, far off along the edges of the paddy fields, refusing to be forced to rest. It was during this time that there were pounding sounds that could be heard from the narrow room tucked away in the back of the house, a room known as the **charte**. This room belonged to the younger women of the family. It was here that they spent their afternoons grooming each other, gossiping out of Grandma's earshot, sharing each other's love stories and speaking in grandiose fashion about their husbands' scandalous bedroom behavior. This room also served as the workspace where they performed tedious tasks, such as milling the rice and other grain or preparing tapioca, fruits, and other vegetables for drying in the sun so that these precious foodstuffs could be preserved for the coming monsoon season. Most importantly, this was the room where the young women gave birth to new members of the family.

> *I was told that I was born in this back room before the midwife could arrive, several weeks earlier than my time. No one could tell me how early, but they did tell me that I was quite small. No one weighed babies then, so I have to take these eyewitnesses at their word. Grandma was present and, of course, in charge. As the story is told, she wrapped me up in a soft white cotton cloth and kept me in in a wicker basket, underneath the mango tree, in the early morning sun, for several hours daily, for the first month or two of my young life. This set up constituted nature's incubator keeping the baby warm and comfortable while it's fragile body harvested the healing energy of the sunbeams.*
>
> *My own children would arrive decades later, across the ocean, in the heart of the New World, during my medical residency in Chicago. They, too, were premature, but both of them would spend many days, not under a mango tree, but, rather, in the neonatal ICU, neatly packed away in high tech incubators, hooked up to oxygen monitors, IV lines and feeding tubes. Thankfully, they both survived this ordeal and continue to live healthy productive lives.*

On the back wall of the **charte**, close to the floor, was the forbidden entrance, a small, rectangular, three by four foot door, a foreboding barrier that, when accessed, led to the mysterious and wondrous cellar. When open, one could gaze into the musky darkness of the belly of the house, a place where seldom-used heavy tools, earthenware, large cooking utensils made of stone, brass and copper, and grandpa's fishing and farming essentials were stored. Only adults were permitted to enter this catacomb, and they did so only before weddings, funerals, baptisms, or big feasts in order to collect those items needed for that particular event. Grandpa, of course, also entered this room periodically, retrieving his cherished implements and proceeding on to whatever venue he felt needed his attention.

As children, we were forbidden to enter this underworld full of mystery and intrigue. Primordial, fear-inspiring ghost stories of all colors and textures emanated were from this cellar, including one about a gold link chain, weighing several kilos and supposedly hidden in its deepest recesses. Legend had it that this gold was recovered from the family's drinking well by one of the ancestors when it one day came up in the bucket along with the water being drawn. This gold, however, was never to be seen or touched, as it was cursed, guarded zealously by the specter of the ancestor who first found it, but who later lost his mind and committed suicide by jumping into the very same well from which the gold had been retrieved.

Apparition or not, at least once every summer at this ancestral home, we children managed to crawl into the cellar, hearts pounding, as we hoped to catch a glimpse of the beam of golden light that would escape its hiding place and see it for ourselves. Of course, after only a few seconds of peering into the musky darkness and conjuring up images of diabolic ghouls and goblins brushing against our skin, we raced out of there with some demonic phantasm in hot pursuit of our sanity. These forbidden forays also took place during the quiet, sunny afternoons when everyone and everything, including the hens, cows, dogs, flora and fauna seemed to be resting, lulled by the cooling afternoon breeze that flowed in from the flooded paddy fields.

On one side of the very same multipurpose room stood the **Oral**, an upright, granite mortar that stood two to three feet high, and which was used for milling and pulverizing grains, mostly paddy. The main ingredient of **Idiyappam** consisted of this hand-pounded, reddish-brown rice powder. The paddy (unhusked rice grain) would be placed in the mortar, and two women, one on either side, would pound the grain by skillfully throwing a long cylindrical wooden pole, tipped with a heavy cast-iron cap as pestle, rhythmically into the mortar one at a time. We children would beg the aunts to let us have a turn, and once the technique was mastered, we would delight in the dance-like movement that was required to pound the grain. Following a short period of pounding, the husks would separate and the contents of the mortar would be taken into a flat reed receptacle called a **moram**. The aunts would then go through the ritual, rhythmic shaking of the contents in the **moram**, periodically throwing it up into the air in what appeared to be an almost effortless act, until the husks separated from the grain and landed in different parts of the **moram**). The reddish-brown rice grains from the de-husked paddy would then be placed back into the mortar, to be pounded to the desired smooth and grainy consistency needed to make **Idiyappam.** This powder would be put through a sieve and then be roasted on a low heat in a heavy, flat, large brass alloy *Urli,* until the sweet, nutty aroma of roasted rice announced the forthcoming serving of **Idiyappam** for breakfast the next morning.

The next day the women of the household woke up early and set up trays covered with banana leaves, in order to make the little Bird's Nest Rice Noodles. The dough kneaded in hot water would be squeezed in handheld, brass noodle presses, flowing, thin, shiny, white noodles, gently placed over small mounds of grated coconut, so as to make little bird's nest shaped noodle mounds. These works of art would then be placed in copper steamers lined with banana leaves then steamed to perfection. The little savory Birds Nests would then be arranged in the *morams* lined with banana leaves once again until ready to be served steaming hot, with mutton, egg or horse gram (small brown chickpeas) curry, made in a coconut sauce.

Coconut Stuffed Birds Nest Rice Noodles
Idiyappam

Equipment needed

Steamer (bamboo or metal), or **idli** steamers & handheld noodle press (available in Indian stores or via internet).

Ingredients

1 kg finely ground roasted rice powder, or **Idiyappam** mix, available in some Indian Stores

Boiling water as needed

1-2 cups fresh or frozen grated coconut

¼ tsp cumin seeds

Salt to taste

Banana Leaf if available (may substitute parchment paper)

Process

- Place rice powder in a deep dish.
- Add salt to taste and mix thoroughly.
- Pour boiling hot water in a slow stream, and mix vigorously with wooden spoon until a dough-like consistency is achieved. As the dough cools, knead it with your hands, and add additional powder, if needed, to get the dough to the consistency where it does not stick to your hands.
- Place sections of banana leaf or baking paper on steamer shelf. If using *Idli Steamer,* brush surface of steaming pockets with a little coconut oil, and place directly into steamer without banana leaves or baking paper. This is the easiest way to make these noodles.
- Pat down a small dime sized piece of dough, six inches apart, on the banana leaf or baking paper.

- Mix grated coconut with cumin seeds ahead of time.
- Place 1-2 tablespoons of grated coconut with cumin over the dime-sized dough patties.
- *Optional: May add 1-2 tsp of brown sugar to the coconut if sweet noodles desired.*
- Fill noodle press 3/4 way with dough.
- Use hand held noodle press to press noodles around and over the coconut mounts to make little Birds Nest like noodle mounds 4-5 inches in diameter.
- Steam for 10-15 min.
- Remove from steamer.

Serve hot with mutton, egg, horse gram, chickpea or vegetable curry all of which can be made using the same recipe by precooking and substituting the eggs with the main ingredient.

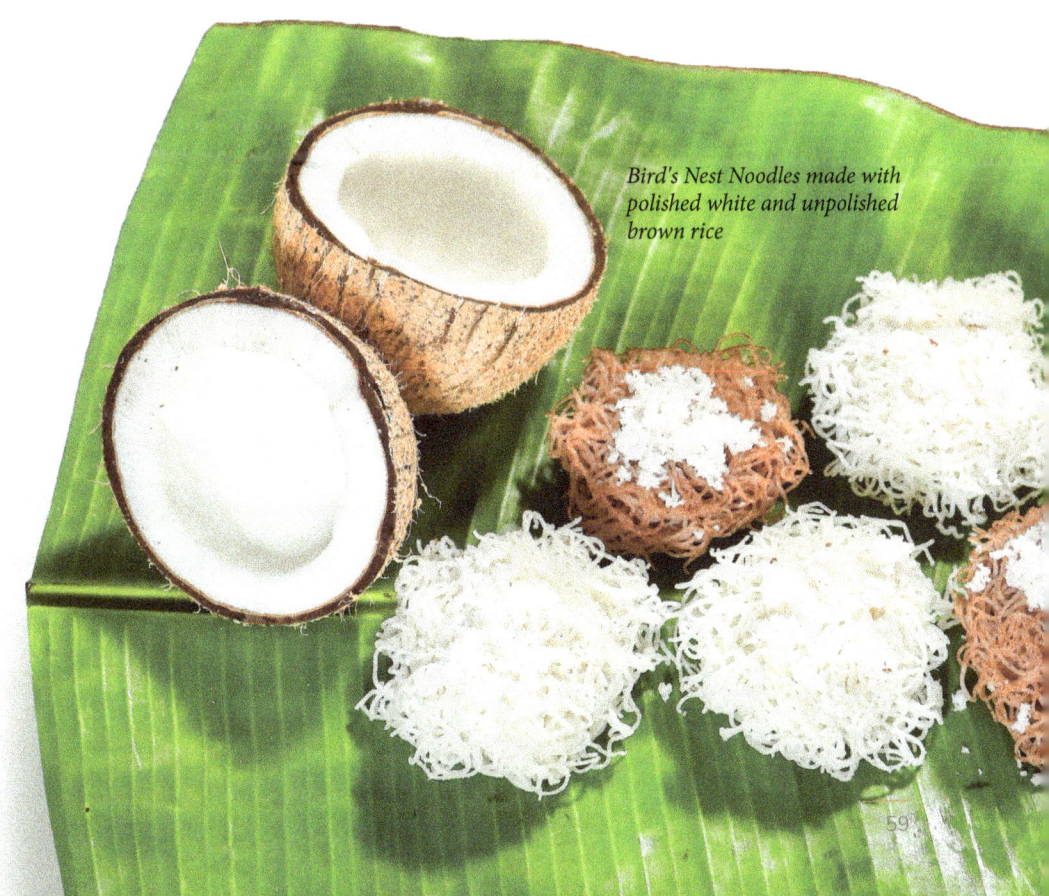

Bird's Nest Noodles made with polished white and unpolished brown rice

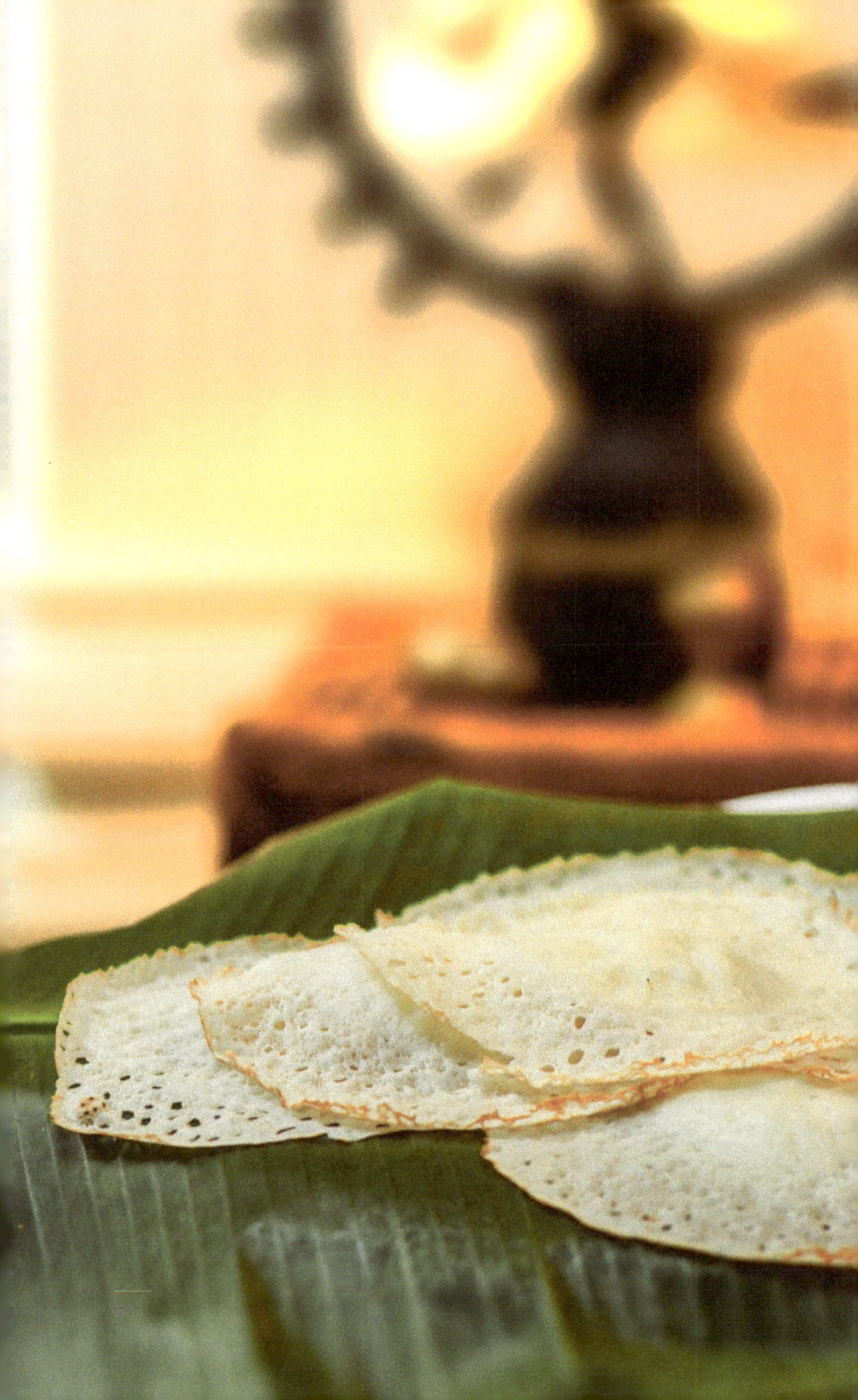

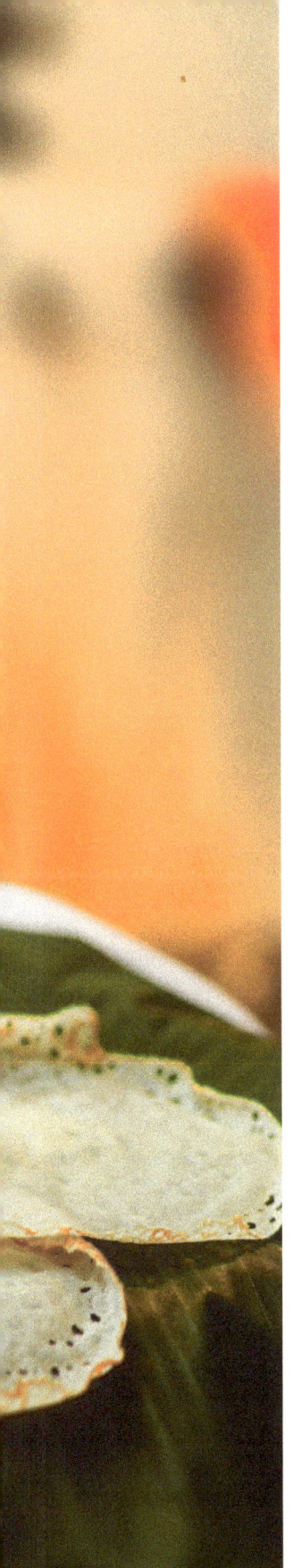

BREAKFAST, BRUNCH AND OTHER MEALS

KERALA CLASSIC FERMENTED RICE CREPES
Appam (Palappam)

A**ppam**, or fermented rice crepe, is unique to Kerala and sports two of Kerala's predominant food sources, rice and coconut. It draws its distinct flavor from the addition of ***toddy***, made from the sap of the coconut tree and lightly fermented into an alcoholic beverage that is heartily consumed by locals. With the passage of time and the decreased availability of unadulterated, ***toddy*** it has now been replaced by beer or packets of yeast, all of which are readily found in general shops throughout Kerala.

Growing up, eating ***Appam*** conjured up holiday memories, special celebrations like baptisms and the arrival of far-flung family members or revered guests. Whenever Grandma and her brood started preparing ***Appam***, it was a foregone conclusion that family, friends and fun were not too far behind, eager to luxuriate in the warmth and hospitality of the ancestral home.

In those days, rice was soaked by Grandma a day in advance, steeping overnight, then ground by hand the next day in a granite mortar. Grandpa, accompanied by an assistant who was specially trained in climbing the tall coconut trees, set forth in the early morning to collect the coconut sap. Alternately, and on days when such forays were not possible due to heat, rain, or the periodic hangover, the two would groggily set out together for the ***toddy*** shop, returning later in the day with the freshest batch of high quality ***toddy*** money could buy. This precious purchase had not yet fermented at all, to ensure the dough would not become too sour, or perhaps only slightly as was ideal for use in the ***Appam*** recipe. During my teenage years and as Grandma grew older and less involved in the household activities, the younger generation of aunts and daughters-in-law would send out the rice to be ground at the local mill. They would then use the resulting rice powder instead of going through the tedious process of grinding the rice at home.

Freshly collected **toddy** (**elam kalle**) was thought to have medicinal benefit and was considered to be an excellent tonic for the young and older alike. We children were therefore invited to imbibe a small glass of what would be an otherwise forbidden drink. In that moment, we felt privileged and honored that the adults would cross such a line, taking the risk of introducing us to this drink, which has been the bane and downfall of many thriving Kerala families for decades.

The abundance, affordability and ease with which the raw materials could be historically procured, made **toddy** the local alcoholic beverage of choice. In its untainted form, and taken in moderation, it was perhaps one of the most naturally occurring, locally plant-sourced, benign, and to some extent, healthiest liquors around, and one which allowed farmers and laborers, who worked hard in the fields all day, to relax, soothe their bodily aches and pains. It had the ability to help them, for a time, forget about the worry and uncertainty that followed each of them around as a constant companion, often allowing a handful of uninterrupted, blissful hours of dreamless sleep. Yet, as human nature would have it, at least one person per Kerala household succumbed to the drunken demon, thus dragging families down with them, and leading to tragedy, discord and a loss of one's already meager assets.

Our beloved Grandpa Varkey was a perfect example of the unsettling role that **toddy** could play in disturbing the peace, tranquility and innocence of childhood. Grandpa was physically engaged in the grueling work of planting banana trees on family property, tending to delicate vegetables that needed frequent attention, trimming trees so as to avoid overgrowth and rot. He supervised workers in the paddy fields who mercilessly roasted in the burning noon and late day sun just to make sure that most of the food needed by the family would come primarily from the land.

As the sun would begin to set, turning the skies pink and heralding the cooler onset of evening, Grandpa Varkey would complete all his tasks for that day and head home. It was not uncommon for him to end his day by casting his circular fishing net, employing one round sweep of his elbow, and filling his copper pot with as many fish as were needed to feed his family a sumptuous dinner that very same evening!

Following lengthy and solemn evening prayers, including the rosary and a litany of novenas, the meal, consisting of steaming mounds of parboiled rice served over a banana leaf, soaked with the gravy of a hypnotically aromatic coconut and tamarind fish curry, would be served. No sooner had it been placed in front of our waiting eyes would it be lapped up in mouthwatering handfuls by all present. Then, with bellies warm and content, we would move on to our next favorite activity.

The best place to sleep for the children who had gathered in the ancestral home during summer vacation was on the gravel courtyard where the expansive reed mat, used for paddy drying, would already have been spread in anticipation of our sleeping arrangements for the night. The children would advance to the back room, where smaller individual reed mats and pillows were stacked. Each child would grab his or her favorites, then scurry to the courtyard to find their favorite spots on the mat, as close as possible to their favorite cousin. Grandpa stationed himself centrally, in the middle of the big mat, reclining lazily on his traditional easy chair, with a cup of spiced tea in hand, brewed especially for him by Grandma, who always kept a large pot warming over her hearth. Grandpa was tall and dark with skin that was sunburned and cured by daily outdoor labor, an extremely thin fellow, every sinew in his body defined and pronounced, and not an ounce of fat to be found anywhere on his lithe and leathery frame.

With all the youngsters filled to the brim with food and happiness, the time had come for Grandpa's ghost stories! First, however, each of us craved a sip from his teacup, which gave off an otherworldly and mesmerizing aroma, if only because that sip came from the edge of his cavernous, alabaster, porcelain bowl, or **Koppa**, from which he drank. This soothing beverage, brewed from black pepper, cinnamon, anise, and cloves, boiled and then sweetened with molasses, was a welcome tonic, soothing Grandpa's aches, and taking care of his nagging cough, which came from exhaustion and his **beedi**, or locally rolled tobacco, which he habitually smoked during his work breaks. After each one of us had had his or her sip, we parked ourselves around Grandpa's chair, impatiently anticipating his forthcoming, spooky narrative. We were never disappointed. Grandpa made it a point to tell these stories as if they had happened to him personally, and, as children, we believed that he was the hero, standing tall, acting bravely, and remaining undaunted in the face of terror and peril.

One of Grandpa's best and most thrilling stories involved an immense figure, human in form, but much taller, even taller than the highest coconut tree. This creature—one with no discernible name—appeared on several occasions, mostly in the same place, almost always near the bend in the river that flanked Grandpa's paddy fields. Grandpa considered its appearance to be an omen, often forewarning of illness or death in the family, or of an upcoming flood or crop blight. Grandpa, however, was crafty and had his wits about him, and he knew the solution to this tremendous form of danger that lurked in his midst. All he had to do, at the moment when he felt most compelled to glance again, was muster all of his inner strength and avert his gaze from the creature's visage. This herculean feat certainly and miraculously saved more than a few of his friends and family from an unspoken and horrible fate! He also made it a point to mention that he would recite the verses of St. George (known as **Giwargis Sahado**, dragon slayer and saint of the Orthodox and Catholic traditions, revered among the Keralan Christians) in order to contain and dispatch the fiery fiends that could harm the family, neighbors and crops.

Another tale that he reveled in sharing involved a dismembered forearm, replete with hand and fingers and bent on inflicting revenge on the miscreant who had perpetrated certain crimes. As this yarn neared its climax, the hand would manifest in our mind's eye, sneaking up behind us and grasping the napes of our necks, ready to choke the life out of us! With gleeful and chaotic screams, we would flee into the verandah, securing ourselves behind nooks, crannies, chairs and doorways. When a few minutes had then passed without incident and when our racing hearts had calmed down, we would once again run outdoors and flop on the mat around Grandpa, eager to receive the rest of the story.

After Grandpa retired, we were all still excited, riled up, and unable to sleep. We would lay on our mats, wide awake and staring up at the starry sky, taking in the magnificent sight of the vivid and sparkling swirls of the Milky Way. The clarity of this heavenly landscape felt close and palpable. At times it simply felt as if we were right there with those celestial bodies, space travelers, visiting luminous and blindingly beautiful, faraway places, at one with these distant points of light and the universal life that emanated from them.

Finally, and after a day of playful abandon, lovingly-served, marvelous, and hearty meals, and nurturing flights of fantasy, complete with frightful ghosts and cosmic castaways, our heavy-lidded eyes would close in the wee hours of the morning. We would have probably slept throughout the night, and well into the middle hours of the morning, so exhausted were we from our extended and ebullient bout of familial fanfare, were it not for being woken up by a sudden and unexpected downpour that would send us scrambling for cover. Half asleep, we all piled into the verandah, holding the mats over our heads, and hugging our pillows for protection from the elements, then falling asleep once again on our makeshift mattresses, our weary but sated bodies buoyed by the support of the cool, windswept terrace.

There were some unpleasant times as well when Grandpa would venture into town to purchase provisions for the family. These were times that would fill those of us possessing discerning hearts with a mild to moderate sense of dread and unease. This vague and nagging fear would stem from Grandpa's penchant for stopping on the way home to visit one of the **toddy** establishments along the river. It was there that our normally reserved and proper patriarch would give himself over to some demons lurking within, and drown some of his unexpressed sorrows and doubts situated among those of similar ilk. Inevitably, he would arrive home inebriated, irritated and impatient, drunkenly going on at length about his difficult brood and his increasingly hard life.

Grandpa's state of mind during these alcohol-fueled tirades spilled out in loud, fearsome monologues, going on at times about his own father's or wife's shortcomings, how he often felt shortchanged, and how we did not appreciate him for all the good that he did. During these spells, he would defer from joining us in evening prayer, and the hoped-for fish curry was woefully absent from the dinner table. The children, disappointed, but wary of arousing Grandpa's ire, went to bed inside the house, subdued and nonplussed. Thankfully, it was most fortunate that these were rare occasions. They did, however, puncture our innocence with the sharp, jagged reality of human suffering and frailty.

On those mornings when full-scale preparations for the **Appam** feasts were under way in the kitchen, we were often woken up by the sometimes atonal but often melodious singing of the mynah and cuckoo birds, as well as the loud cawing of crows, who, sensing heavy activity in the kitchen, would excitedly announce the imminent arrival of guests. We would quickly jump up, unceremoniously aroused from slumber and join in the celebration of the upcoming feast, swooning as we inhaled the sweet, nutty aroma of *Appams* being cooked over the hot, cast-iron, dome-like woks. We sniffed greedily as the smell of the egg curry or mutton, infused with a tantalizing bouquet of Malabar spices, reached our noses, tickled our palates, and sent us spiraling into yet another round of joyful revelry!

> Prepackaged, ready-made, dry **Appam** mixes, complete with yeast and other familiar ingredients, are now available in most Indian grocery stores so that, once again, those who live in the diaspora can take, with great convenience and ease, the requisite and desired shortcuts and participate in the illusion of recreating the culture, context and ritual associated with the authentic recipes that were handed over to us by our forebears.
>
> Sadly, these well-intentioned but poorly executed attempts to recreate the taste, nuance and substance of the original dishes, using ingredients that are processed into lifeless, machine-made concoctions, result in tragically disappointing outcomes, leaving one endlessly yearning for the people, customs and traditions that were once such a salient and essential touchstone in the lives of those fortunate enough to have lived through that experience. Even more than this though is the lack of the one most important ingredient of all: the "love" embodied in the cooking and all that came with it. This is what truly matters, and this is what is truly and indescribably lost.
>
> As a society, we have embraced physical convenience at any cost, thereby rejecting the "ingredients" that are essential to a viable and life-affirming existence: love, attention, appreciation, and the hard work, effort and challenges that must be encountered in order to forge a lasting and meaningful human bond. "Convenience," wedded to the enabler of "mass production" and born of a desire for unnatural and unhealthy wealth accumulation, has created a witch's brew of discontent and disconnection; it is a distorted and dysfunctional potion that is slowly but surely poisoning and killing us, in mind, body and spirit! Only the "inconvenience" of love can give birth to joy and meaning, and this is true whether we are talking about conversation, caring, or recipes. It is all truly part of one big picture, and that tapestry needs to be one that is woven with the human heart at the center of its expression.

Kerala Classic Fermented Rice Crepes
Appam

Ingredients

2 cups white rice (basmati, jasmine, or plain), soaked as instructed below

1 cup grated coconut

1 tsp packaged yeast or 4 ounces of beer

¼ cup cooked white rice (separate from item #1)

1 tbsp sugar

Salt to taste

Water, 1-2 cups as needed, to grind rice to a thin, liquid batter

Appam cooking dish is available in most Indian grocery stores

Process

- Wash thoroughly and soak rice overnight in enough water to cover about 1 inch above layer of rice.
- The next morning, scoop rice out with a ladle and grind in a blender or food processor. You may need to do it in 1-2 batches to be able to grind the rice optimally. Add water to the blender slowly while grinding to produce a silky batter that will pour easily.
- Add sugar, yeast or beer to above batter and let ferment overnight.
- The next day, cook 1/4 cup of well-washed rice, adding 1/2 cup of water. Cook on high heat until boiling, then cover and simmer.
- Grind the grated coconut and cooked rice in blender with enough water to make a loose paste.
- Mix the above paste into the fermented batter, add salt to taste and mix thoroughly, and wait for 30 minutes.
- Heat the *Appam* dish over high-medium heat until hot, then pour one medium-sized ladle of dough into the middle of the dish. Quickly pick up the dish by the handles and swirl the mixture around to add a lace of circular dough around the middle pool of the dough, then lower heat and cover with lid provided for 1-2 minutes, making sure the middle thicker section is cooked and the surrounding dough is crisp and lacy.
- The *Appam* should peel off the dish smoothly and with minimum effort.

- Lay cooked **Appams** out on a large open tray and serve hot or warm. Do not cover until completely cool (condensation can soften the **Appams** and make them pasty if covered while warm).

Serve with egg, mutton or mixed vegetable curry.

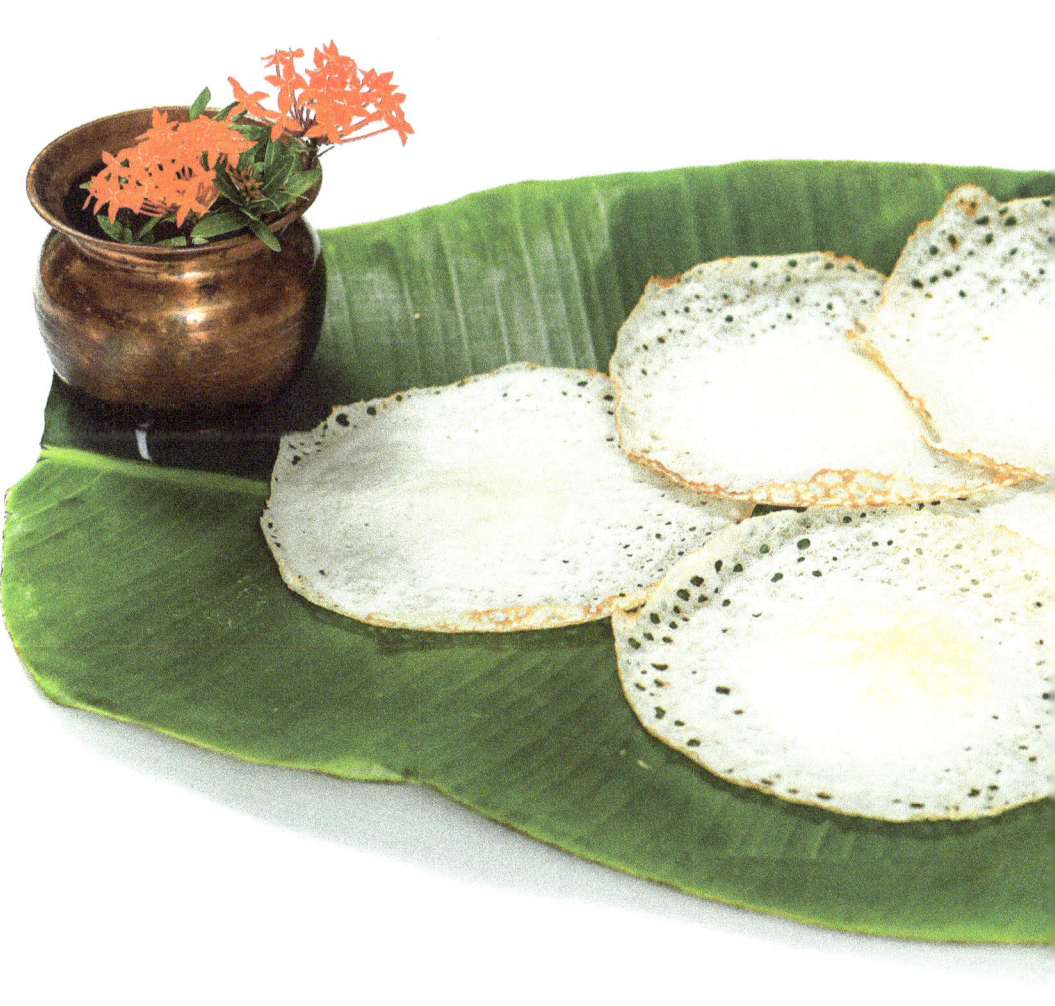

RICE AND LENTIL CREPES AND BUNS
Dosa and Idli

I had been introduced to *dosa* as a young child in Kerala, but my intimate relationship with this classic Southern Indian recipe began after I adjusted to life in the United States.

I met my future husband when I was a freshman at Marquette University in Wisconsin. A whirlwind romance led to marriage six months later. His Hindu Brahmin family background made the whole affair intriguing and exciting. Brought up in a very traditional, Keralan Catholic family, I found Hindu culture to be complex and mysterious. My Jesuit teachers piqued my interest more when I took a course in comparative religions. As a result, and when we married at this young and impressionable age, I was suddenly immersed in learning about Brahmin culture and cuisine. This led to my early exposure to *dosa*.

Dosa is an ancient recipe that is mentioned as early as 1000 AD, and also appears in a 12th century AD Sanskrit encyclopedia. The modern version of *dosa* is thought to have originated in *Udupi*, a small town on the southwestern coast of India, in the state of Karnataka. My husband's Brahmin ancestors from *Udupi* had, for the first time, uprooted themselves and moved away from their roles as priest farmers. They became traders, businessmen and professionals in urban cities including the city of Mumbai, formerly known as Bombay.

Brahmin men traditionally served as Hindu priests. They were the only ones who had access to the inner sanctum where temple deities resided. These holy men were considered pure and trained to perform the sacred Hindu rituals. Tutored from their teenage years onward, in Hindu monasteries called *Matts,* this elite group was groomed to carry the secret rituals, chants and were the only citizens privy to this powerful and secret knowledge. They are believed to be endowed with the knowledge and skill to elicit energies that could change fate already set in motion by the movements of the planets. Traditionally well-versed in the sacred texts, chants, rituals, astrology and **Vastu** (the science of accurate living space construction and arrangement to harness or avoid the positive and negative energies of the Universe), they presided over every auspicious and inauspicious event in a Hindu family's life. For example, using astrology and mathematics, they were taught to create and interpret horoscopes. Then, by linking the time of birth to planetary positions, they predicted an individual's destiny. Next, they guided the individual to a more fortunate or safer harbor through recommendations that included rituals, prayers, fasting, gemology, yoga, and many other techniques that were thought to have the power to mold and change energy.

> *This migration of the Hindu Brahmin priests signaled the first step in the journey of the caretakers of the **Spirit** (at least symbolically) from the otherworldly to the worldly. This led to an erosion of spirituality and the ascendancy of materialism. The Hindus prior to that time understood that suffering was a tool to sharpen the spirit, until its light shone so brightly that it blended with the light of the Creator and one did not have to be reborn. In other words, it was a way to pay off one's karmic debt from the previous life and move on to higher life. However, these customs also resulted in great social injustice. They fostered and rationalized the injustices of the Hindu Caste System that pervasively lead to extreme mistreatment and disrespect of human beings in the lowest class of the Hindu Caste System, the Shudras, who performed menial and "unclean" tasks for society like cleaning toilets, sweeping the gutters etc. With each rebirth, the soul apparently had to keep paying off the Karmic debt in suffering. Society rationalized the plight of this lower class by considering it inevitable to the individual's Karmic debt.*
>
> *Now, in this brave new world, there could be only one reason for suffering—one's own lack of resourcefulness. All one had to do was to keep moving until status and financial freedom had been achieved. At this point, one might imagine that happiness was inevitable. Alas, the pot of gold called "fulfillment" that waited at the end of the rainbow remained empty, as the inevitability of death and the anxiety of separation from the material world became paramount.*

Over the century, the caste system in India disintegrated, leaving traditional roles and diets behind. The people have drifted to places within India and abroad, adopting the culture of the new cities and lands that they now inhabit. Most are no longer vegetarian. A significant number have abandoned their traditional rituals and forms of worship, embracing modernity wholeheartedly both in India and abroad.

The Brahmins were treated with godly respect, and, as such, were permitted certain liberties. It is well known that the Brahmins, though vegetarians, loved to overindulge in rich foods, especially **ghee** laden treats.

As one would expect, food played a central role in this culture, and my husband's family of origin was no exception. His mother, grandmother, and aunts planned and prepared meals that enchanted and delighted. Their talents and skills were considered to be their birthright. From this community, in the late 1950s, was born the quintessential South Indian classic, the **Udupi Restaurant**. Now ubiquitous in most Indian cities, it serves original Brahmin vegetarian recipes from **Udupi** of which **Dosa** takes centerstage.

The preparations for **Dosa** are not simple. From stories my husband told me about his childhood, Amma (my mother-in- law) soaked the rice and **Urad dal** (lentils also known as **Black Gram**) on the morning prior to the meal. On the evening of the same day, she reportedly flopped herself down on the floor, and positioned herself smack in the middle of the hallway of her small two room flat in Mumbai. Here, she set about performing the laborious task of grinding the dough for the **Dosa.** This scene was made more comical by her four children frequently surprising her and skipping over her to get across the room, causing her to loudly proclaim her consternation and displeasure.

For hours at a time, Amma would grind the rice, then the lentils, moving the large, heavy, oval, granite pestle around the hollow carved out center of the larger, circular, granite mortar. Her hands, a flurry of continuous motion, danced to and fro, one constantly moving the pestle held in the cup of her palm in a circular motion, the other directing the smooth, silky dough back into the belly of the mortar. Once this part of the process was complete, and the contents had been securely placed in a deep steel vessel, she raised herself from the floor in an amusing series of fits and starts, calling the household to aid her in transporting the heavy dish to the kitchen counter, close to the stove where it would ferment until the next morning. The fermented dough would then be ready to be made into crisp, papery **dosas**.

> *Amma has now graduated from her ancient grinding stone. Now her maid makes the dough in minutes in redesigned granite lined steel grinders with electric motors. It is remarkable that granite is still maintained as the grinding surface for these large unwieldly modern electric devices. Of late she too purchases the premixed dough in neatly packed plastic bags at the local grocery.*
>
> **Urad dal**, *when ground, makes a sticky, starchy paste. This paste was used in making casts for fractures in India just as recently as a few decades ago.*
>
> *As I reflect on this period of my life, with its innocence and uncontrived beauty, I find myself mourning the loss of yet another cog of what composed this integrated existence that is lacking in contemporary life.*

Amma's **dosas** were famous. Her generosity was well known to her Mumbai neighbors in the ancestral building in which she lived and to those outside the family as well. My husband's school and family friends were just a few of the fortunate recipients of her cooking. Everyone knew that the first and last batch of **dosas** cooked were reserved for the perpetually hungry cricket-playing, Judo-savvy son who later became my husband. Accompanied by his colossal, youthful appetite, he demanded a special place and preferential treatment in Amma's kitchen.

Over the years I observed Amma's skill first hand during my visits to Mumbai, and later, in America. After priming the cast iron **dosa** griddle with **ghee**, she spread the smooth, velvety dough onto the pan with impeccable skill. Then, as the crepe approached readiness, she sprinkled more **ghee** on the **dosa**, and then flipped it over. In a few seconds, out came the crispy, thin treat, folded at the end of her spatula. Coconut and mint chutney completed the picture, and the hot, crispy, savory, scrumptious morsel was quickly and summarily devoured.

Dosa

Ingredients

(Makes 4-6 *dosas*, depending on size)

⅓ cup **Urad dal** with or without skin.

⅓ cup white rice (Rice to **Urad dal** proportion is 3:1, increase quantity for servings)

½ tsp fenugreek seeds

Salt to taste

Process

- Wash and soak rice, **Urad dal** and fenugreek seeds together in 3-4 cups of water.
- After 6-8 hours, extract the grains from the water and grind in blender in small batches as the grinder will tolerate, adding only enough water to make a liquid paste like pancake batter.
- Keep overnight in a warm place, such as the inside of the oven without turning on the heat or near the stove. (*This mixture ferments overnight and does not need refrigeration. In very hot climates it may need to be tasted and refrigerated if the dough starts to get too sour*)
- The next morning, add salt to taste and enough water as needed to make the mixture a consistency that will slide off spoon without difficulty.
- Heat a non-stick or cast iron **dosa** or pancake griddle, also called a **tawa.**
- Season the surface of griddle with 1 tsp of **ghee** or oil of choice.

- Pour a medium-sized ladle full of dough (about ¾ cup) in a circular motion to swirl from center outwards to cover most of the surface of the griddle, spread gently with the base of a ladle to make a thin crepe.
- In few minutes, sprinkle a few drops of **ghee** on the surface of the crepe and, using a fine spatula, flip the crepe. Leave on low to medium heat until crispy.
- Fold into two. Or place a 1-2 tsp. of **Potato Masala** in the middle and fold over from either side. Serve hot with coconut and mint chutney or sambar.

Drizzle with honey to make a sweet and savory treat.

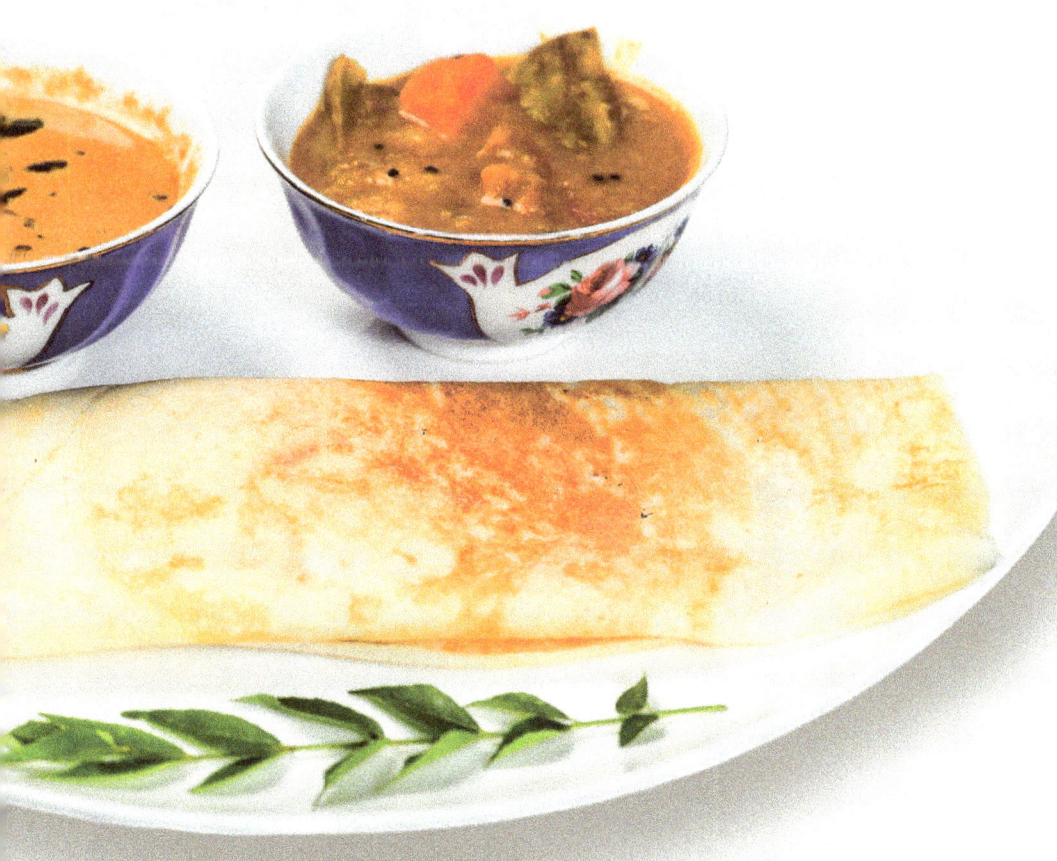

Masala Dosa with Coconut Chutney and Sambar

 **Idli**

The same dough as above can be used for **Idli**.

Follow the same procedure as above but reduce the water and grinding time for a thicker, coarser dough.

You will need an *idli* steamer available in Indian stores or on-line.
- Boil two cups of water in an *Idli* steamer.
- While water is boiling grease the *idli* molds with ghee, butter or any oil of choice.
- Pour batter into the molds, leaving enough room for the buns to expand.
- Place the molds in the steamer and steam for 8-9 min (can use a tooth pick to confirm the buns are cooked). No residue will be left on the tooth pick after piercing the buns if they are well cooked.
- Grease a butter knife or teaspoon with oil and gently extract each bun from its mold.

Serve hot with Coconut Chutney or Sambar.

Recipes for coconut and mint chutney and sambar can be found on pages 162-163

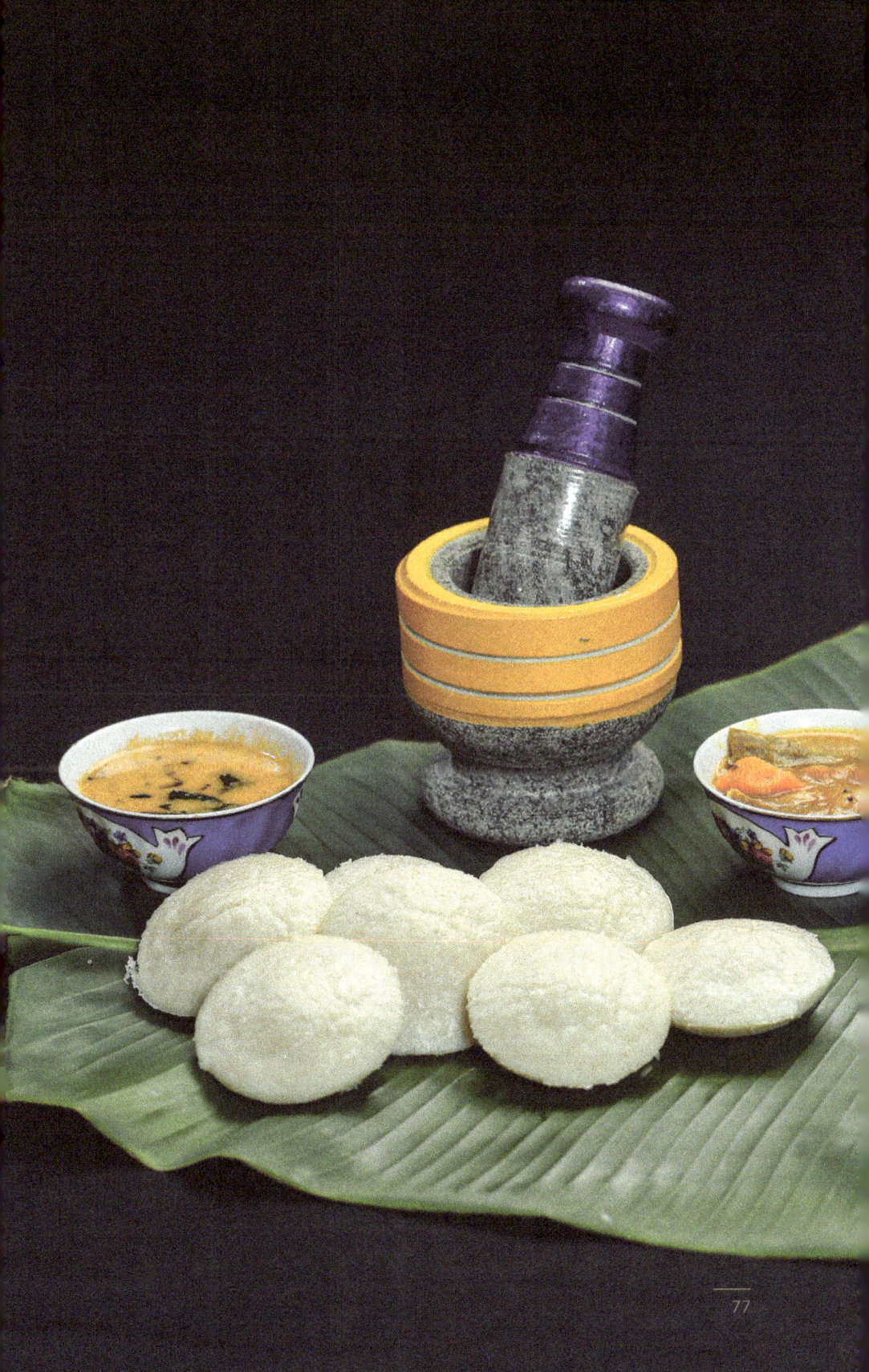

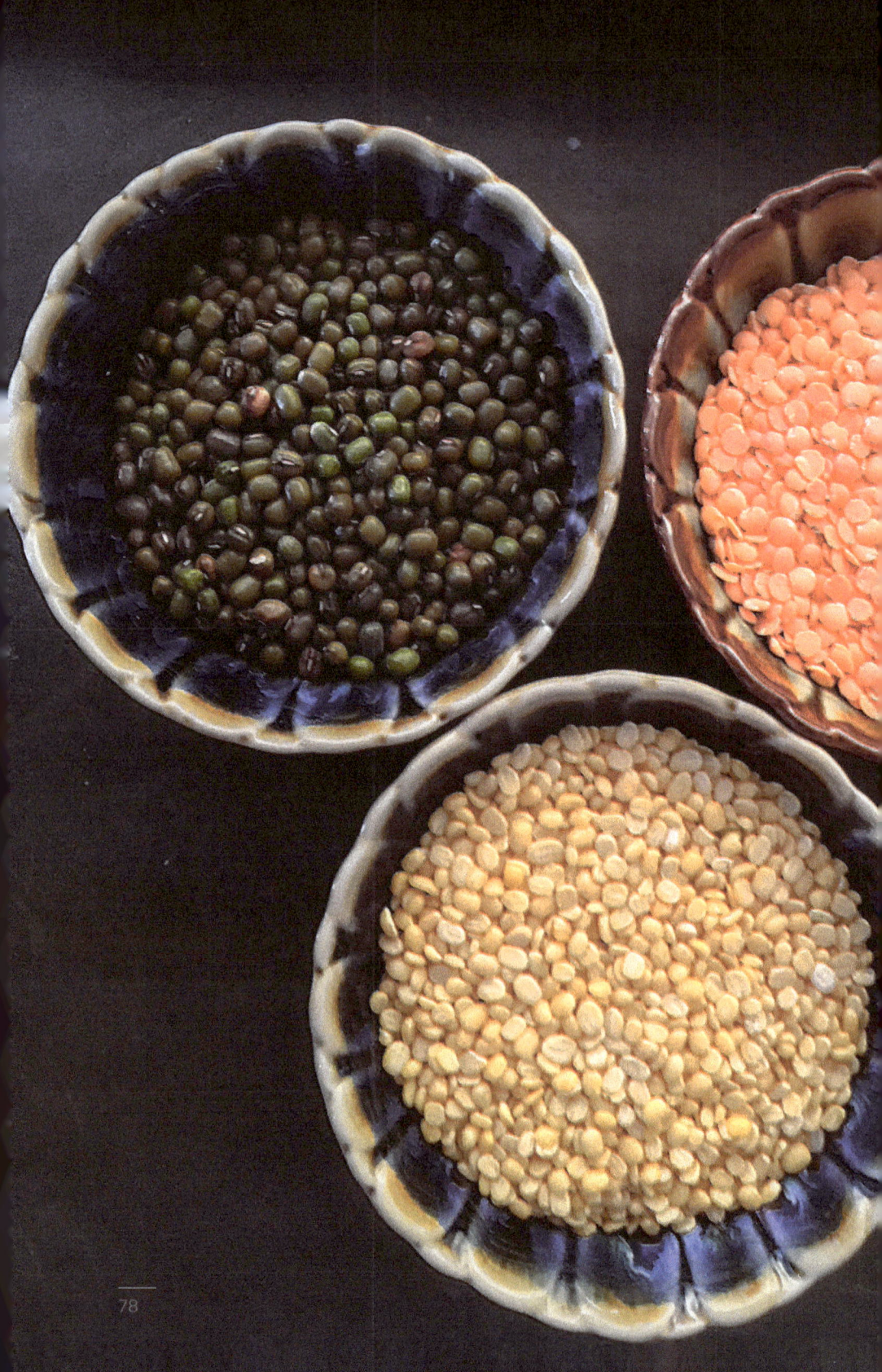

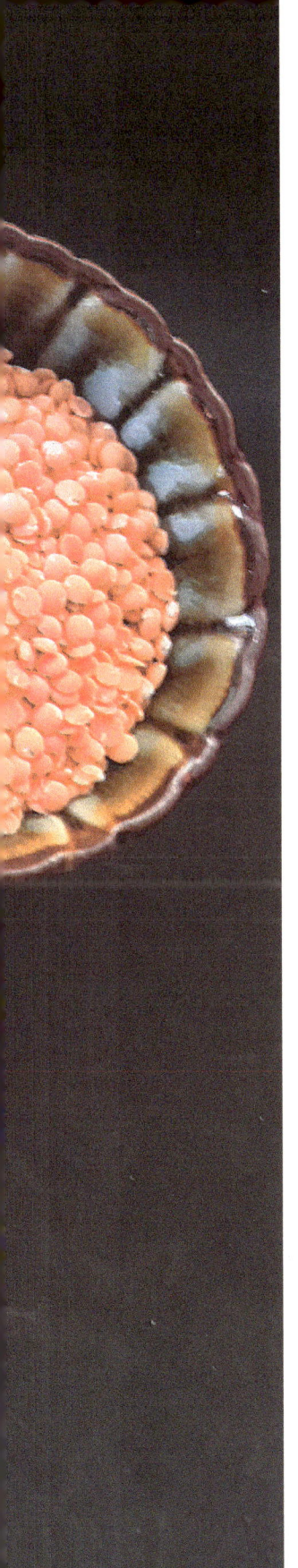

CURRIES AND LENTILS

GRANDMA'S SUNDAY EGG ROAST CURRY
Motta Curry

Grandma Teresa could always be relied upon to fall back on her scrumptious egg curry dish whenever the menu called for a hearty source of protein, especially when a meat curry, which would pair perfectly with like Appam was not affordable. These occasions typically arose on a Sunday, a day for brunch, when a non-vegetarian dish showed up as part of menu when the family returned from Mass or when an unexpected guest arrived, and there was no time or resources to prepare a meat dish.

Several yards away from the ancestral home, at the edge of the backyard, was the chicken coop. Grandpa carefully constructed the coop from bamboo, covering it with coconut wood in the form of a trellis, thatching it with woven coconut palm leaves, and then finally spreading hay for the floor. It was only during the evenings that the chickens would head toward the coop and finally come to rest after a long day of barnyard bustle. From dawn until dusk, the roosters, followed closely by their harem, roamed the property, scratching for worms and insects and making their presence known with their clucking and occasional loud arguments and fights, establishing their pecking order with authority and pomp.

Grandma's day would be punctuated periodically by the insistent and loud clucking of the hen after she had laid her egg. The entire family, including the brood of visiting children, was well attuned to this signal, and an egg hunt enthusiastically ensued. The chickens most often did not use the chicken coop to lay their eggs as they preferred the little caves they had carved out beneath the dome-shaped haystack. At other times, they could be found lazing in the cellar or *Ara* occupying a cozy corner where the used gunny sacks were stored *Ara is* a large, wooden, room-sized chest in the heart of the typical Kerala house and around which the rest of the dwelling was constructed.

Grandma knew each member of her feathered friends by name. At meal times, once a day, when she would scatter rice or wheat kernels as a tasty morsel for the hens, she made it a point to call each one by name….. *Tresiammm..ae… Marykutty..ae*….making her own telltale, cackling sound as part of the feeding ritual. Once in a while, when one would not show up, she would recruit us children to undertake a search. Curiosity periodically turned to tragedy when a trail of feathers would signal that the missing bird had become a fox's meal. These crafty creatures were known to slink in from the neighboring paddy field. We were all attuned to their devious ways and unwanted and uninvited incursions.

Easter, Christmas and New Year's were days of sacrifice for Grandma and her feathery brood, and one or two of her "children" would have to be offered up for the holiday feast. In her heart, Grandma knew which ones would be chosen, and despite her reserved and calm, outward demeanor when feeding her babies, her resigned and pensive look betrayed the trepidation in her heart. We all knew, with great and penetrating clarity that Grandma preferred making Egg Curry to Chicken Curry.

Grandma's Sunday Roast Curry
Motta Curry

Ingredients

1 dozen medium, boiled eggs, peeled and carefully sliced in half length wise (*Grandma used a sewing thread to cut the eggs after they were peeled, and it worked remarkably well*)

1 medium, red onion, sliced finely in circles

1-2 tsp of crushed or grated fresh ginger root

6-8 cloves of garlic, chopped or crushed finely

1 tsp cumin seeds

1 stick of cinnamon

4-5 cardamoms crushed, with or without discarding the pod skin

2-4 cloves, whole

1 tbsp fennel, roughly crushed

½ tsp turmeric powder

¼ tsp chili powder, increase or decrease based on taste desired

¼ tsp black pepper

1 tbsp coriander powder

2-3 dashes of Asafetida

10-20 fresh curry leaves or ½ cup chopped fresh can substitute with cilantro leaves

1 tsp of rice vinegar or regular vinegar

1- 2 tbsp coconut or olive oil

1 can coconut milk

Salt to taste

Process

- Heat oil in low-med heat.
- Place cumin seeds in oil for 30 sec.
- Place onion, ginger, garlic, cardamom, cinnamon stick, cloves and curry leaves into the mixture and sauté in low-medium heat until onions are caramelized golden brown. *If using coriander leaves instead of curry, use it as instructed at the end of this recipe.*
- Lower heat and place coriander powder in the mixture. Mix on low heat for 1-2 min.
- Add chili powder and half of turmeric and stir for 1-2 min on low heat.
- Add salt and black pepper.

- Add 1/2 cup of water to the mixture, mix, and heat on low heat for 1-2 min. Stir gently every 3-4 min so that the mixture does to stick to the bottom of the cooking dish.
- Turn off heat.
- Pour 1 medium can of coconut milk and gently place the eggs into the mixture taking care not to break the eggs apart.
- Add fennel, asafetida and more salt to taste if needed and mix ingredients gently by swirling the pan while on very low to medium heat.
- Place the eggs carefully into the sauce with a serving spoon. Place the eggs with yolk facing up so that they do not crumble into the sauce.
- Increase heat for 1-2 min then turn off heat.
- Pour vinegar over the top of the curry. Do not mix.

After 2-3 min, sprinkle coriander leaves on top if using coriander leaves instead of curry leaves

Serve with bread or starch of choice, like wheat chapati (tortilla), pita bread, naan or Appam.

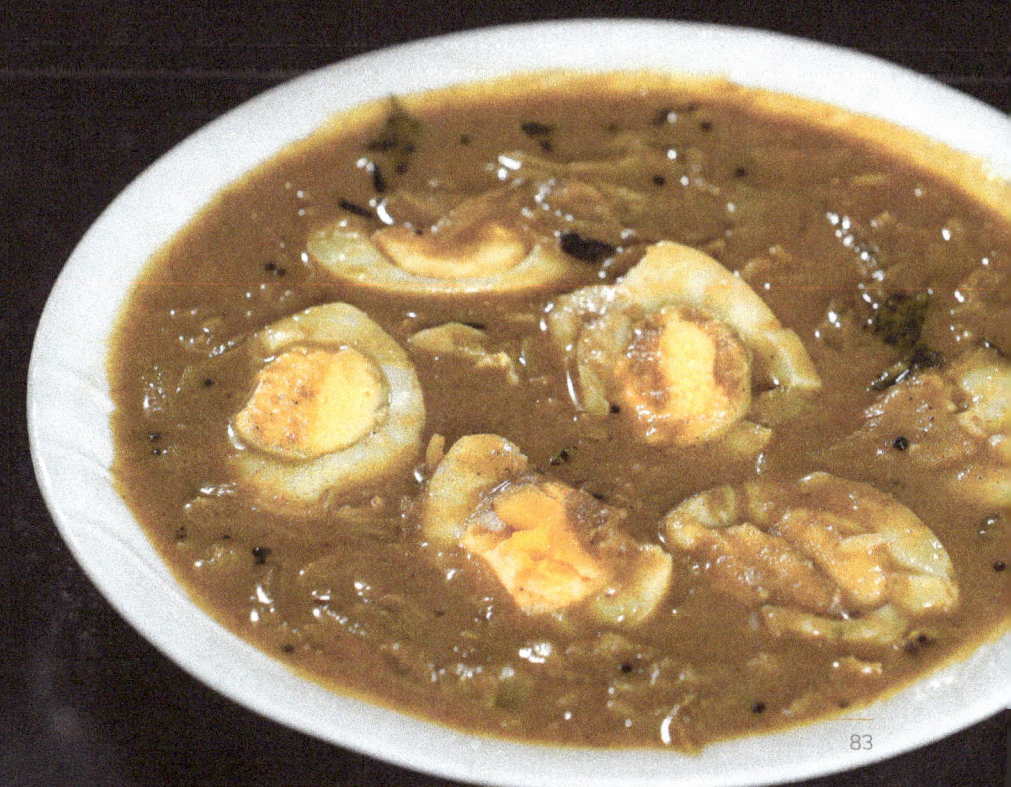

KERALA STYLE COCONUT FLAVORED DAL
Parippu Curry

Lentils (*Dal*) of numerous varieties have been a staple food of India since historical times. **Toor, Chana, Masoor, Urad Dal** and **Mung Dal,** which in the past two decades have become very popular in the West, have fed millions in both the opulent and meager kitchens of India. With a good mix of protein, carbohydrates, fiber, vitamins and micronutrients such as folate, thiamine, potassium and magnesium, **Dals** have kept populations alive in India for centuries.

Throughout my young life in northern India, **Dal** dishes such as **Dal Tadka** *(sautéed Dal), dal* with various vegetables like spinach or mustard was an integral part of our daily fare. A South Indian version called Sambar, that has tamarind added is a version that pairs perfectly with rice and various South Indian dishes. The ubiquitous use of **dal** could be attributed to its affordability and availability.

Dal is intrinsically linked to a panoply of remarkable childhood memories due to an incident that occurred during my pre-teen years in Jabalpur, in central India where we lived. At that time, both my parents were in the army, and we lived in an army containment area where the raising of cattle or any form of livestock other than chickens was forbidden. This had no effect on my determined and creative mother, who insisted on harassing my father long and hard enough to build a hidden cow shed in the back of the army bungalow to which our family was assigned.

Over the ensuing half dozen years, several cows lived happily in this contraband backyard barn, grazing on vast tracts of poorly patrolled, military pastures. Many families bent this rule, resulting in misfortune for those who were caught doing so. The cows were impounded in far-away facilities, and large fines had to be paid in order to get them back again. Nonetheless, my mother insisted that we take such risks. She was single minded and simply refused any attempts to be convinced otherwise, going so far at times to make life rather challenging for those who failed to see the method to her madness.

It was no easy feat maintaining a mini-dairy on forbidden army property. We had one or two helpers. Young men, who migrated to the cities in search of livelihood, were recruited and became part of our extended family for several years. It was during this time that, once a year, a bullock cart arrived, weighed down with a frighteningly large consignment of hay. The arrival of the farmer and his son, from a village far enough away that several days' travel was required, was heralded as an auspicious occasion.

It seemed that, except for black tea in the morning, most of the day the young man and his father sustained themselves on water alone, which we provided for them in a clay samovar that kept the water cool. They usually worked the entire morning and settled into an afternoon slumber under a Banyan tree in the afternoon, protecting themselves from the piercing rays of the sun that wilted people, flora and fauna alike. Come evening, the men would start their work again, grabbing large bundles of loose hay and skillfully placing them on their heads, securing the bundles tightly with their long, sunburnt, knobby arms. They would then walk to the distant end of the backyard and arrange a haystack around a tree trunk or a pole, making a dome-shaped haystack, impermeable to wind and rain. The process would take two to three days to complete.

When the rays of the sun disappeared into the western horizon and a mitigating breeze soothed the bodies and spirits of these bone-tired souls, they ceased working and turned their attention and actions toward tending to their own needs. Approaching a nearby public tap with their steel bucket, they rinsed off their bodies until a measure of acceptable cleanliness had been achieved, then proceeded to light an oil lamp at their makeshift altar beside the block cart, and lastly joined hands as they recited their evening prayers. This was followed by the care and feeding of the bullocks. Finally, they prepared and consumed their evening meal.

Day after day, the same fare was eaten: a few wheat **chapatis** (tortillas) made fresh daily on an outdoor fire pit composed of three stones or bricks. One could place a utensil over this makeshift cooking surface, the fire under it lit from twigs that had been collected nearby. While the father kneaded the dough for the **chapatis**, his son tended the dal boiling in a small clay dish over the fire. When the meal was ready about one hour later, the father and son would enjoy their meal of **chapati** and **dal,** spiced with salt and an uncooked fresh green chili each, taking small bites of these pungent condiments in between their mouthfuls of food. A supply of green chili seemed to always be at hand, thus ensuring that this meager meal took on grander proportions. Often this was their only meal of the day.

By the time we went to bed, we could still see the dim light from the oil lamp, the father and son squatting next to it, talking softly. I am not sure how or where they slept as they were usually hard at work by the time we woke up the next morning.

Apart from **sambar,** which is essentially a watery, vegetable soup with a very small amount of **dal** added to thicken it, I remember eating **dal** in Kerala only as **Parippu Curry** for **Onam** celebrations. **Onam,** a holiday celebrated by Hindus, Muslims and Christians alike, is a feast unique to Kerala. It is a joyous festival, celebrating the harvest of the preceding season.

Ripe with lore and ritual, during **Onam**, the citizens decorate their courtyards with floral designs created with fresh flowers, and bursting with the colors of the local flora and fauna. This is also the occasion for families to buy new clothes, kitchen and houseware goods and gadgets at the numerous craft markets that open up in towns and villages during this season. Most of the products found at

The hardscrabble existence of the Indian family farmer as well as family farms around our planet has been made even more difficult with the introduction of GMO crops into the world agricultural system. While there are obvious benefits of GMO for crop yields and pest/weed control, the downside is often much greater. Since time immemorial, farmers were able to save some seed crop from their harvests to replant, but after being tricked into using GMO seeds with false advertising of its benefits, they have to use the little money they have to purchase new seeds. This has led to the suicide of hundreds of thousands Indian family farmers yearly, often by drinking farm chemicals.

these markets are locally produced: coir mats, stone and clay cookware, and handicrafts made of coconut shells, wood or palms. On several occasions, I recall vacationing in Kerala and observing children wildly and excitedly celebrating their ten-day **Onam** furloughs from school.

The highlight of this holiday revolves around a feast. Consisting of twenty-one vegetarian dishes served on banana leaves, **Onam** makes it a point to flaunt the produce and the flavors of the Keralan harvest. **Parippu Kari** is a major player on this list with coconut and cumin imparting to it its unique Keralan flavor.

> *Sadly, modern-day school children in Kerala are cloistered in their homes, in front of their computers and books, studying for entrance exams and other school requirements. These all-consuming activities have taken over their lives to the point where a festive occasion like Onam is viewed less as a crucial cultural and social event and more as an annoyance or inconvenience. My heart breaks when I meditate on this notion and I pray that some semblance of balance and an infusion of meaning and inner awareness will one day return to our lives and livelihoods bringing focus of our precious lands and how the food in our plates comes to existence.*

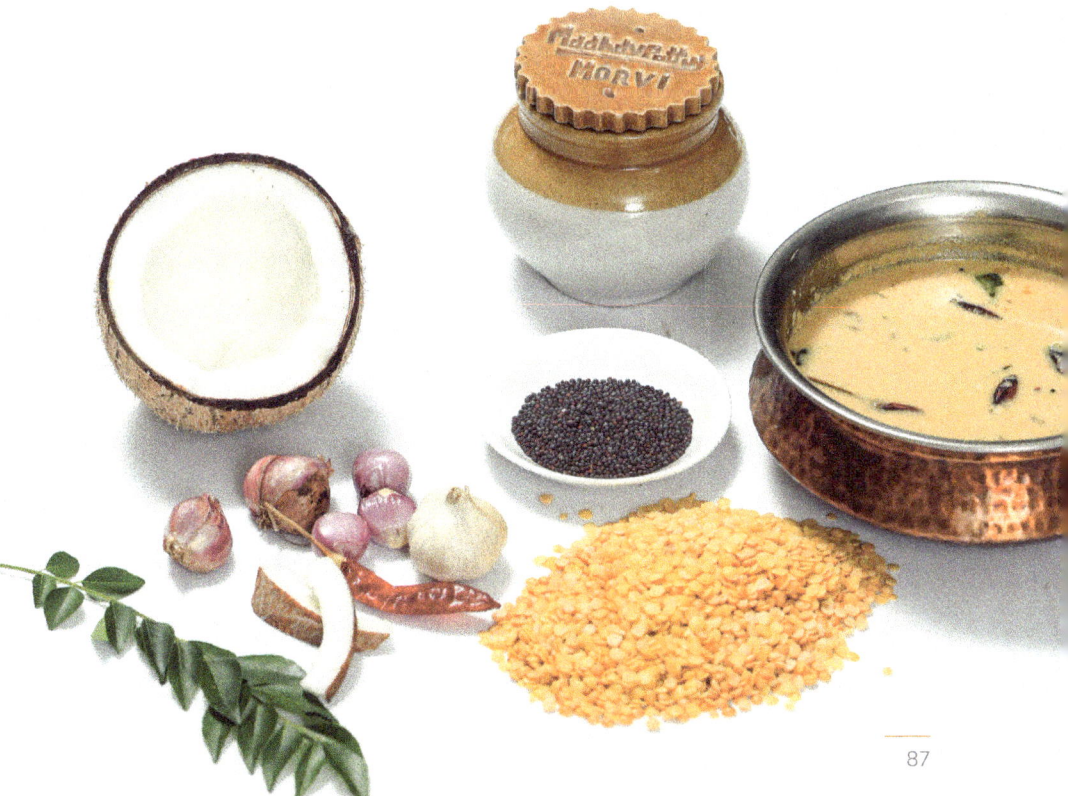

Grandma's Kerala Style Coconut Flavored Dal
Parippu Curry

Ingredients

- 1.5 cup lentil of choice (***moong dal*** is best)
- 1 cup grated coconut
- ½ tsp cumin seed
- 2 cloves garlic peeled
- 1 tsp grated or grated fresh ginger
- ½ tsp turmeric powder
- 1 whole green chili, sliced partially lengthwise
- 1 tsp mustard seeds
- 1 stalk or 12-15 curry leaves
- 2 dried red chilies, broken in half
- 2-3 dashes Asafoetida
- 1-2 tsp coconut oil or ghee or sunflower oil
- Salt to taste
- 4-5 cups of water

Process

- Wash lentils thoroughly with water and drain.
- Place lentils in a saucepan, add 4 cups of water, and cook on high heat until contents boil.
- Lower heat to medium, add green chili, and cook open on medium to low heat until lentil can be crushed between index finger and thumb.
- Add water, as needed, keeping the cooked lentils in a liquid state.
- Once lentils are cooked, lower heat to lowest setting and keep covered.
- Grind coconut, cumin, garlic and ginger, adding 1-2 tbsp of water until achieving a medium-gritty consistency.
- Add salt to taste, turmeric, and contents of the grinder into the cooked lentils. Mix thoroughly with a wooden spoon. Use a whisk if needed to bring the whole mixture to a uniform consistency.
- In a small frying pan, heat **ghee**, coconut oil, or other oil of choice.
- When oil is hot, add mustard seeds and keep lightly covered, with a gap, until mustard seeds pop.
- Add dry red chili and curry leaves to hot oil, heat for 30 sec, then add 1-3 dashes of Asafoetida to the hot oil and remove from heat immediately. Pour over the prepared cooked lentils.

*Served best with hot rice and **Pappadam** (a fried, paper thin, lentil-based wafer, served as a condiment with any rice dish).*

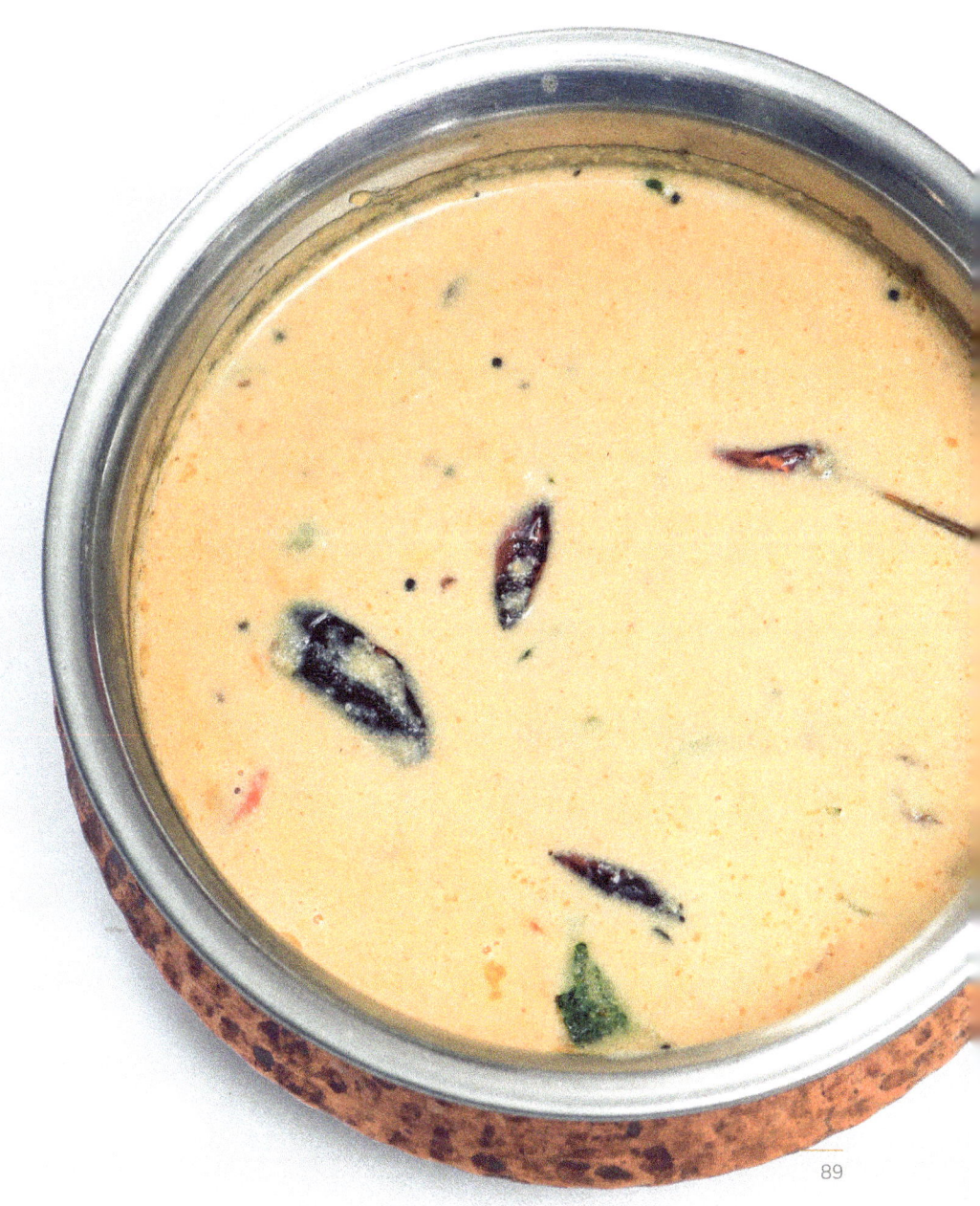

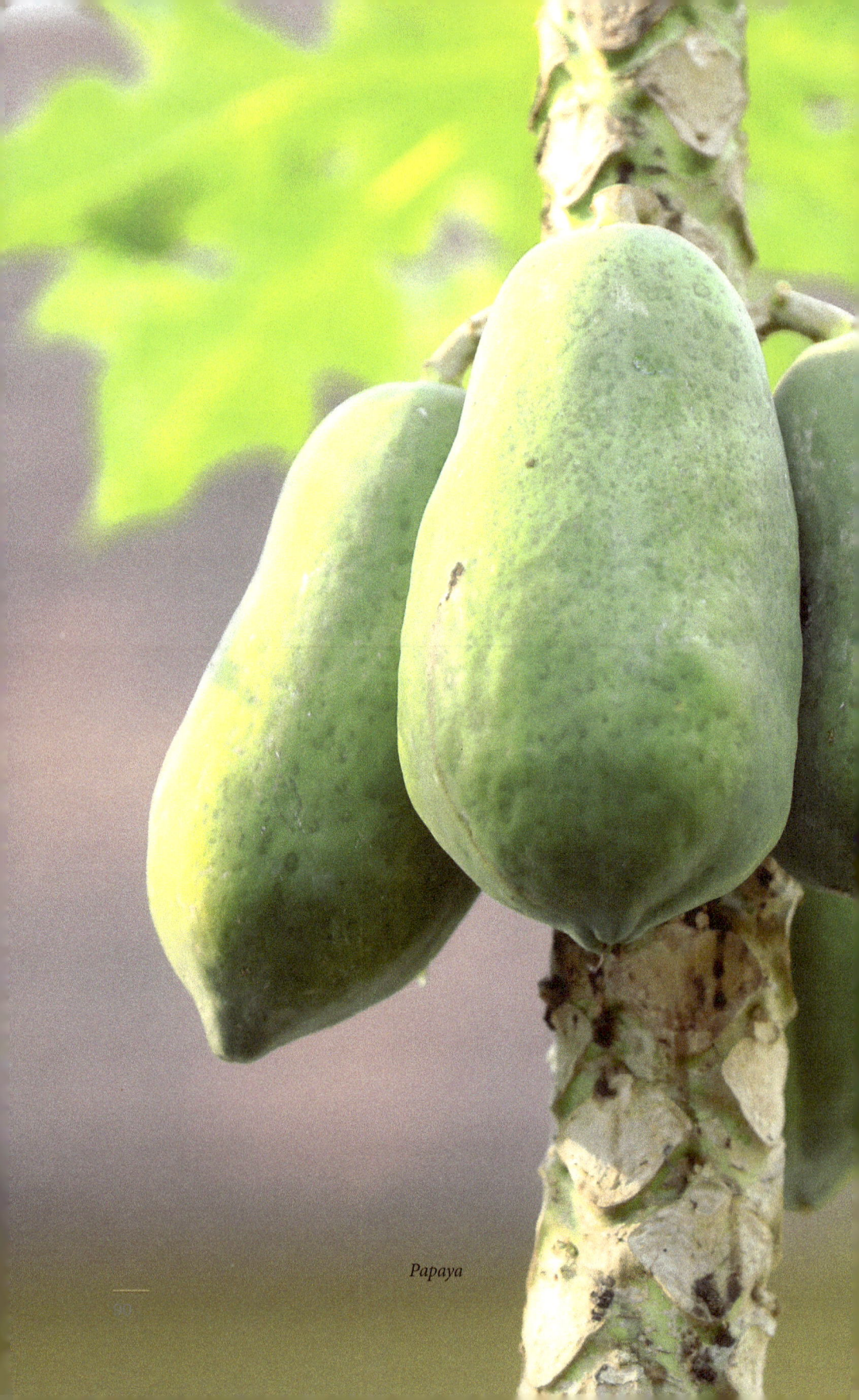

Papaya

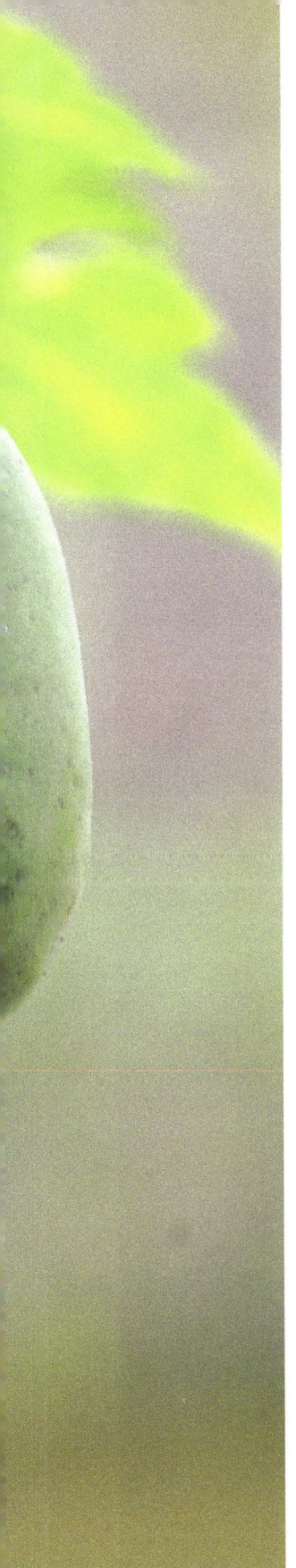

VEGETABLES

RAW SAUTÉED PAPAYA
Kapalanga Toran

P apaya plants were abundant in the lush, tropical garden surrounding our ancestral home in Kerala. Seeds were sown year-round and willy-nilly by birds of all feathers, who feasted on the sweet, pulpy flesh. These plants appeared in the most unexpected locations: in the middle of the courtyard, sometimes near the edges of the house, in the middle of vegetable beds, between fruit trees, or wherever the birds happened to alight. It was a symbiotic relationship, a marriage of convenience.

This plant's most notable feature was its tall cylindrical trunk, resembling an electrical pole. This trunk grew rapidly from six to twenty-five feet in height, all in a matter of weeks. Sprays of long-stemmed, elongated, snowflake-shaped leaves fanned out from the end of each pedicle, forming umbrella-like canopies at the top of each plant. Between the leaves, olive-shaped bright green fruit sprouted directly from the trunk on single, ropy stems. The fruit remained green as it grew and morphed into whimsical shapes, including large ovals, elongated with tips turned up like a bird's beak and other fanciful, random shapes and sizes. The disciplined ones produced more uniformly shaped fruit, and harvesters favored these because they were easier to sell.

Once these oval-shaped young fruits were noticeable, it only took a few days for the fruit to grow to full size and for the tropical sun to soak into the fruit's green skin, coating it with a yellow-orange glow signaling that the pulp inside, now a salmon-orange color, was ripe. Each ripe fruit when cut dripped with sweet aromatic juice, a healing libation loaded with many remedies for just about everything.

Harvesting the fruit from the top of the tall trunk required special skill, as the trunk was not strong enough to allow the homemade ladder any reliable support. As such, a long stick, skillfully manipulated at the base of the stem, ensured surgical precision in the harvest as well as prevented any damage to the cluster of fruits hanging in tight proximity around the current fruit being harvested. If one were especially adept, the free hand would catch the fruit as it fell, precluding it from getting bruised on impact with the ground below.

As I remember, Grandpa was the only one who could pull this stunt off. He then turned his precious catch over to Grandma, admonishing her to deal with his precious cargo in a respectable manner. Grandma's Papaya recipe focused more on the unripe ones, the ones with green skin and raw flesh. Known as **Kapalanga Toran,** this dish stands out in memory as one of great satisfaction.

Kapalanga Toran appeared when the days were hot and dry, when the vegetable harvests were few, when water was scarce, and when no special guests were expected. This recipe popped up frequently on the menu during the Lenten fast. Meat and fish disappeared during this time, in the months of April and May prior to Easter. For this season, known for its solemn and quiet, contemplative days, this humble dish with its inviting nutty flavor and chewy texture was appropriate and welcome.

Dubbed the poor family's staple, yet loaded with digestive enzymes, antioxidants and immunity-boosting substances, this recipe promoted a degree of weight loss and clarity of mind and soul.

Sautéed Raw Papaya
Kapalanga Toran

Ingredients

1 lb papayas, peeled and with seeds removed, then roughly grated

1 cup grated coconut (available in most Indian grocery stores in the freezer section), or ½ cup dried coconut flakes soaked ahead of time for 10-15 min in 2-3 tbsp of water

½ cup white onion, roughly chopped

3 cloves of garlic, thinly sliced

1 tsp crushed or finely grated fresh ginger

1 green chili, cut in the middle, or 1 dried red chili pepper broken in half (optional and based on desired spice level)

1 tsp mustard seeds

10-15 curry leaves whole fresh or dried

½ tsp turmeric powder

½ tsp fresh ground black pepper

3 pinches or dashes of asafetida*

Sea salt to taste

1-2 tablespoon coconut or other oil (coconut or sesame oil preferred)

Process

- Heat oil in a medium sized skillet, flat pan or wok. Be careful not to burn oil

- When oil is hot, drop mustard and cumin seeds, curry leaves and dried red chili pepper in oil (make sure heat is adjusted so that oil is not smoking). Cover loosely with air gap or mesh until mustard seeds pop.

- Lower heat to medium and mix in onion, ginger and garlic into the oil.

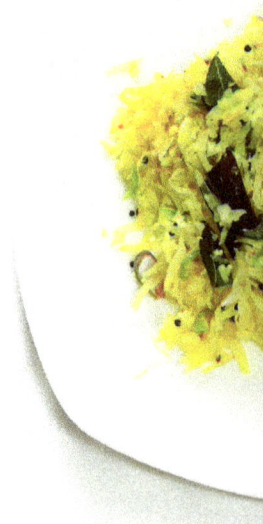

- Sauté until onions slightly brown.
- Mix in chili powder and asafetida to mixture.
- Turn heat down to very low and wait 30 seconds.
- Add grated coconut and papaya, turmeric, salt and pepper. Mix thoroughly, using two wooden spoons, making sure the mixture does not burn at the bottom.
- Blend all ingredients evenly, then pat to form a flat compact mound and cover with tight-fitting dome to avoid condensation.
- Raise heat for one minute, then lower to very low setting for two to four minutes.
- Open lid and cook for one to two minutes, stirring frequently (overcooking changes the flavor and consistency).
- Remove from heat

Best served hot with rice and golden spiced buttermilk or bread of choice.

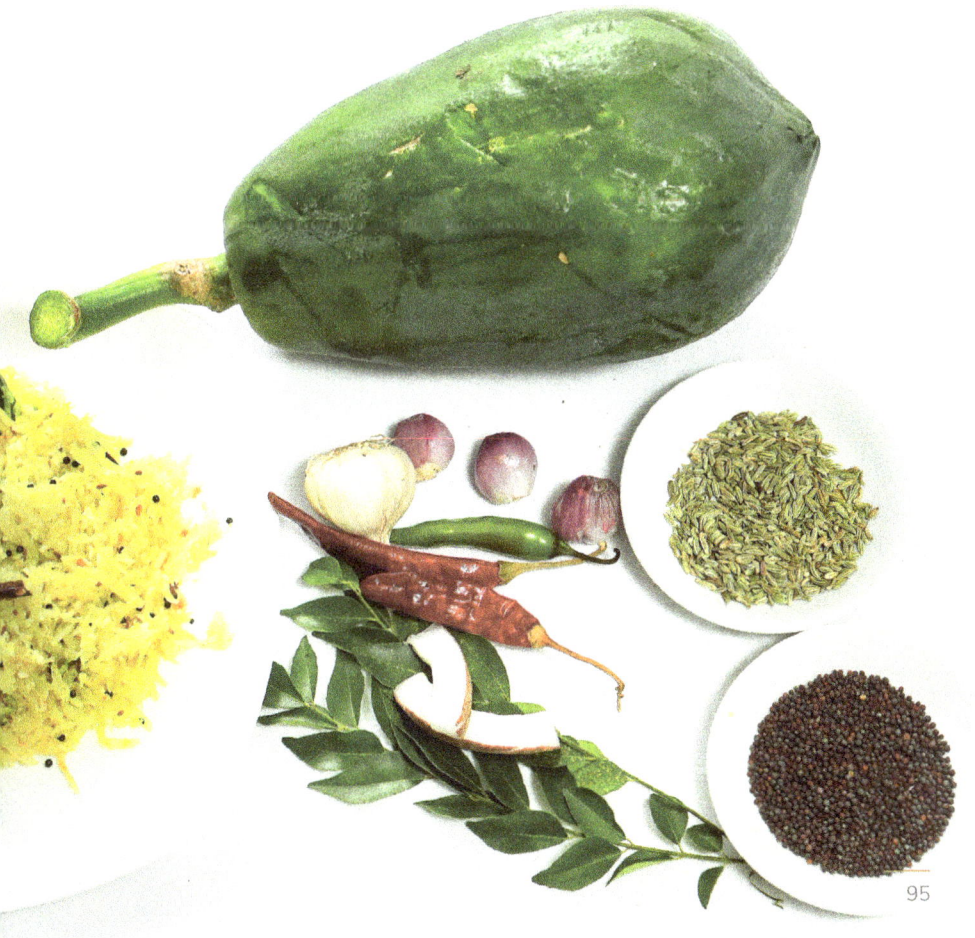

GRANDMA'S CHINESE STRING BEAN SAUTÉ
Payar Mezhukkupuratti

Vegetables harvested from the ancestral land were plentiful, beautiful and remarkably tasty. Grandpa single handedly managed to grow them. The women and youth of the house were responsible for harvesting them. Chinese string beans, bitter gourd, okra, eggplant and snake gourd were some of the many vegetables grown. With the exception of the monsoon season, vegetables took their turn, sprouting and maturing throughout the year.

Long, crisp, verdant Chinese string beans, called ***payar***, were the household favorite. Delivering a savory, nutty flavor and conveying a mild sweetness when young, these legumes lent themselves to various permutations of Keralan cooking. They grew twelve to eighteen inches in length and, when harvested at the appropriate time, were crispy and could be broken into smaller pieces by hand. At other times, the local women knew how to skillfully dice them into thin flakes, holding them over their index finger with great precision, speedily slicing them into paper thin segments, using foreboding locally crafted raw iron kitchen knives. I have seen that skill only in Kerala.

My fondest childhood memory of these beans is of the children who visited during the summer holidays. They could not resist raiding the crop. The long, shimmering specimens hung down in strings, usually from tapioca stems or stick trellises six or more feet high. We walked silently through the vegetable patch or tapioca fields and picked the beans, enjoying their superbly crunchy taste. We were forbidden to do this, and it was never a good idea to elicit Grandma's wrath. If she did not have enough of the crop remaining for the preparation of a dish that she was planning, heads would roll.

If the yield was generous, the last harvest would be left on the plants to mature and dry, and the seeds would be removed for storage as dried beans for use at a later time. Some of the seeds were saved, carefully tied up in cloth bundles, and stored in reed baskets that hung in an outside shed for planting for the next season.

> *I remember, years later, hurriedly rushing to purchase string beans when I first saw them in the United States. I was shopping at the Indian grocery store on Devon Street in Chicago. The beans seemed longer and coarser and I was unable to break them apart with my fingers. Moreover, the skill with which I could dice them on a cutting board was far inferior to the skill of the women of my ancestral home.*
>
> *I tried to recreate the recipe but had to leave out the coconut pieces as I could not find them ready-made in packets at the Indian grocery stores. I lacked the tools or skills to work with a whole coconut at that time. Happily, the dish still tasted better than all the other vegetables I had become used to in America.*
>
> *Years later, when we had purchased our first home in Illinois, the fact that I was doing my medical residency did not deter me from planting my own vegetable garden. I remember spending mornings of my days off in the garden with my young children reliving my own childhood. These beans became one of the vegetables that I regularly planted. To my great pleasure and surprise, the hot, humid Chicago summers produced robust and bountiful crops of beans in eight to ten weeks. My mother, who had historically grown a thriving Indian vegetable patch every summer in her tiny backyard behind her row house in Brighton Beach, Brooklyn, provided me with the seeds. Yes, the seeds were original, and their beans were mouthwatering and crisp.*
>
> *I later discovered that my mother, with her incredible green thumb and single-minded determination, recruited many of her neighbors, most of them immigrants from India (especially Kerala), as well as from Kashmir, Pakistan, Guyana, Russia, Georgia, Uzbekistan and many other countries. They took turns helping her with her garden. Mother gladly returned the favor, sharing her largesse of Chinese string beans, bitter gourd, eggplant, okra, and other tropical vegetables with those fine folks. A retired Registered Nurse, she was my inspiration and mentor,*

a woman of tenacity, courage: a trailblazer who brought our family to the new world. She taught me to plant my own garden, employing tried and true techniques from her homeland to ensure a handsome return. It became my turn to share the result of my efforts with my neighbors in my new home on the other side of the country. They were delighted and surprised as they marveled at the exotic vegetables with their unexpectedly luscious flavors.

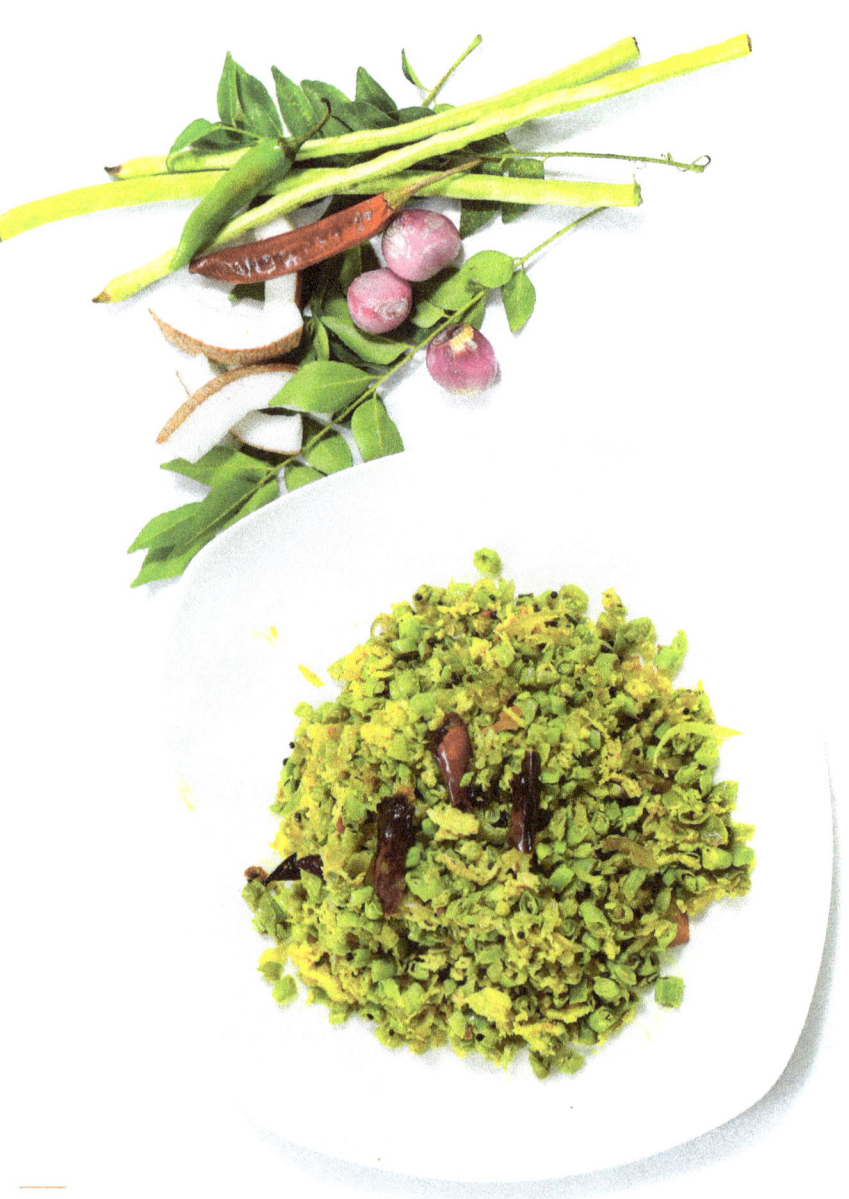

Grandma's Chinese String Bean Sauté
Payar Mezhukkupuratti

Ingredients

- 1 pound Chinese String Beans cut into 1-1.5 inch pieces
- ½ medium sized red onion cut into long slices
- 5 garlic cloves peeled and diced in long slivers
- 10-15 curry leaves, fresh or dry if available
- 1 green chili whole, sliced in the middle once (optional)
- 1 tsp mustard seed
- ¾ tsp cumin seed
- ¼ tsp red chili pepper
- ½ tsp turmeric powder
- 2-3 dashes Asafetida (optional)
- 1-2 tsp coconut oil or oil of choice
- Salt to taste (may replace salt with 1-3 caps of Tamari Sauce for even better flavor)
- Coconut sliced in small bite-sized bits (optional)

Process

- Heat oil in a large flat saucepan.
- Place cumin and mustard seeds in oil and keep on low heat until mustard seeds pop. Cover lightly with mesh lid or other lid with slight opening to release condensation.
- Place onion and garlic in the oil. Keep on low heat, stirring constantly.
- When onions are caramelized, add chili powder, turmeric, asafetida, and coconut, and heat for 1-2 minutes, stirring constantly.
- Add 1-2 pinches of salt to the sautéed mixture to taste.
- In a separate dish, add salt to beans and mix thoroughly.
- Add beans to the saucepan.
- Increase heat to high and stir the beans in with the contents of the pan thoroughly.
- Bring the contents toward the middle of pan and pat down with a wooden spoon.
- Cover tightly with a small lid that covers the beans only for 2 minutes.
- Stir thoroughly and lower heat to medium/low, and cover with lid as before. Stir every 3-5 minutes
- Cook further for 5-10 minutes, without lid, stirring often to desired consistency.

Serve as a vegetable side dish with any meal. Can also be eaten in a sandwich, in tortillas, or with rice.

MUNG DAL STIR FRY
Cherupayar Thoran

Each month, Grandpa made trips to the Changanacherry *Chanda*, a market that flowed out from the mouth of the town's boat jetty. Situated about five miles from the ancestral home, the only way to get to this town and its market was to wind one's way through the lazy waterways, traversing a network of rivers and streams called the Backwaters.

Grandpa owned a vast canoe collection with models ranging from those measuring only eighteen inches in width, streamlined and kayak-like in form and features, to substantially larger ones, able to transport entire harvests of rice and seasonal fruits or vegetables to the market. Monthly shopping trips, where only a modicum of goods was to be acquired, were made with the smallest canoe from the collection, which could only be navigated with practice and tremendous skill. Made from hollowed-out coconut trunks and planks of wood from that same tree, these sleek and aerodynamic vessels were held together with fish oil-soaked coir ropes then waterproofed using the same grease. Grandpa had his own canoe-building workshop in the backyard, where year-round he would work for a few hours each afternoon.

After rinsing off in the river and stealing a swig or two of black coffee, Grandpa set out for the market before sunrise. As always he wore his *mundu* for the journey. The traditional attire worn by men in Kerala, a ***mundu*** consisted of a piece of ankle length cloth, tied around the waist and folded in half when needed, to be used like shorts. His chest remained bare, and a white cotton towel, or ***thorte***, sat turbaned around his head, and thus, he would begin his day. Grandpa would step into the canoe, then effortlessly cradle and alternate the oars with melodious precision, the vessel obediently gliding over the waters as if alive, a type of aqueous offspring, hatched from these very same estuaries.

At the market. advancing from stall to stall, he would first sell off his small harvests of seasonal wares such as Chinese string beans, bitter gourd and tubers, eventually emptying his little canoe to make room for the staples needed in Grandma's kitchen that he could not grow himself: lentils, wheat, buckwheat, teas, sugar, molasses, and some spices like cardamom. These spices only grew at higher altitudes at the tail end of the Deccan mountain ranges that, as they descended, seemed to fuse with the Backwaters of Kerala.

These lowland backwaters of Kerala, which are at or below sea level, empty into the Arabian and Indian oceans, connecting with the Bay of Bengal to the west. As far back as biblical times, the disciple Saint Thomas, the Romans, Arabs, Danes and later, Vasco Da Gama, the Portuguese voyager, as well as British seafarers and other seekers and traders, landed on these shores, drawn by the treasures, the land and its rich and swarming waters had to offer.

Grandpa spent the rest of the day unwinding. He would typically start by visiting relatives who lived near the jetty and have lunch and an afternoon siesta in one of the homes. Refreshed and relaxed he then set forth on his return journey, the sky above him a painted salmon, stained by the rays of the setting sun. The chanting from the Hindu Temples filling his mind and heart with primordial reflection and melancholy, something that I too repeatedly experienced during my own days drifting down these rippling byways. Invariably, these ruminations prompted Grandpa to park his canoe at the edge of the river, and imbibe a few glasses of toddy (local alcohol, fermented from the sap of coconut palms) at one of the local watering holes along the river.

Grandpa would arrive home after sunset with his treasures; his mood pensive, his manner quiet and his gait slightly addled. The children knew to carry the procurements noiselessly into the kitchen where the women sorted and placed each item in its designated place. The household was unusually muted on these days, and Grandpa's voice was absent from the evening prayers. The pantry thus replenished our ancestral home would once again see **Cherupayar Thoran** happily appear on the menu.

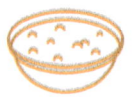

Grandma's Mung Dal Stir Fry
Cherupayar Thoran

Ingredients

- 2 cups **mung dal** with skin
- ½ medium size, red or white onion, chopped
- 4-5 cloves of garlic, crushed or chopped finely
- 1-inch piece of peeled ginger, cubed or finely chopped
- 1 cup of fresh grated coconut
- 1 tsp of coconut oil, olive oil or **ghee**
- 1 tsp of cumin seeds
- 1 tsp mustard seeds
- 1-2 dried red chili
- 1 green chili (optional), whole and sliced partially in the middle 10-15 fresh curry leaves
- ½ tsp turmeric powder
- ½ tsp coriander powder
- 2-3 dashes of asafetida
- 1 tbsp of whole peppercorns
- ½ cup fresh chopped cilantro (optional)
- Salt to taste

Process

- Wash and soak **mung dal** for 2-3 hours and drain in colander
- Add 4-5 cups of water and boil for 10 min, then lower heat and cover, checking frequently until the **mung dal** is partially cooked and making sure that the grains are still firm but crushable between thumb and index finger. Turn off heat and keep open until ready to cook.
- Heat oil in wok or saucepan on low to medium heat.
- When oil is hot, add cumin, mustard seeds, peppercorns, curry leaves, and dried chili. Cover with mesh lid other loose-fitting lid so that mustard seeds do not pop out of the pan.
- Maintain low to medium heat until mustard seeds pop.
- Lower heat and place onion, garlic, ginger, turmeric, green chili in the oil. Sauté for 1-2 min on low heat until onions turn golden brown.
- Add coriander, turmeric and asafetida, and increase heat slightly, sautéing for 1 min on very low heat. Stir constantly
- Add 1-2 pinch of salt and stir.

- Add partially cooked **mung dal**.
- Add more salt to taste and mix thoroughly.
- Add 2-3 tbsp of water, pouring along the edge of the cooking dish.
- Move the contents into the middle of the cooking dish and pat down lightly to make a mound.
- Place coconut in the middle of mound and pat down.
- Sprinkle 1-2 dashes of turmeric and a dash of salt over coconut and pat down.
- Place a lid smaller than the edge of the pan to tightly the contents of the pan.
- Lower heat to very low and cook for 5-15 min, stirring every 3-5 min and keeping covered after stirring.
- Mix coconut into the contents and stir on very low heat. Stir uncovered for few 1-2 minutes to dry off excess moisture.
- Garnish with cilantro and serve.

Pairs well with rice and spiced buttermilk with sautéed vegetables or Keralan fried fish.

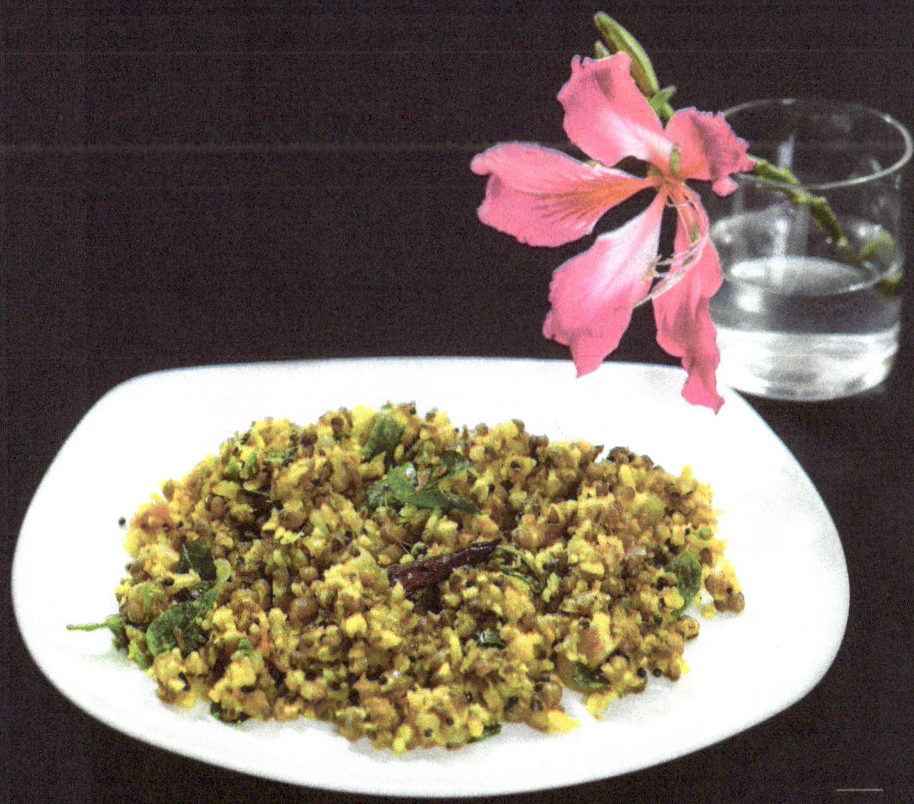

AUNT LILY'S SAUTÉED BROWN BEANS
Vanpayar Olarthiade

Aunt Lily arrived on the scene with a flourish when my mother reached the age of nine. It was clear from the outset that Aunt Lily and my uncle were cut from different cloth. My uncle was a well-mannered and erudite fellow who earned a Bachelor's degree and worked outside Kerala for a pharmaceutical company as early as the late 1950s. With the exception of my mother, who would go on to become a registered nurse, the rest of his siblings had not completed Sixth Form, the British equivalent of high school in those days. When his beautiful bride joined him, everyone was in awe. Aunt Lily was highly educated, had received advanced training in Sanskrit studies, and spoke English fluently. She would later have to turn down invitations from the high school to teach English and Sanskrit because of her domestic obligations. At this early stage of their relationship, they were the pre-eminent power couple of the village.

Now in her nineties, Aunt Lily is still walking, albeit with the help of a walker, speaking English, and reading the newspaper from cover to cover every day. She reminisces time and again about days gone by. On her little study table in her bedroom sits a framed, black and white photo of the newly married couple, my aunt and her beloved husband, on the day following their regal nuptials. Donning a puffed-sleeve blouse and a long gold chain suspended and fashionably hanging down to her navel, she and my uncle resemble those aristocratic characters out of an old post-British era Hindi Bollywood movie. I am inexorably drawn to this photo every time I visit this aging yet timeless woman.

Despite her aspirations to move with her husband to a city outside Kerala, such as Mumbai or Bangalore, and notwithstanding her dreams of becoming a Sanskrit and English teacher, my dear aunt remained confined and ensconced in her ancestral home, a combination of luck and illness in the family preventing a different outcome. She still lives in that same ancestral home, modestly updated to accommodate the needs of modern-day grandchildren. They are IT and medical professionals one and all, scattered to the four corners of the globe, and their visits require a few luxuries unknown in previous eras.

My aunt was unconditional and unreserved in the care and tending of her husband, five children, and in-laws, spending decades tending to their needs, yet never neglecting to hone her culinary skills. My uncle was a demanding type, stingy when it came to compliments, and critical when it came to passing judgment on any food that was put in front of him.

To observe my uncle when he was eating was to be privy to a full-blown comedy show. Frequently opining about too much or too little salt or heat or wrinkling his nose at the unforgivably uneven consistency of the gravy, he resembled a hen clawing around in dirt. He would pick at the food, denuding these artfully prepared dishes of curry leaves, pieces of cinnamon, cloves or black pepper, or whatever he thought he would not like, flicking them off of his plate until it was surrounded by a wreath of spices and edibles that he considered unpalatable.

My aunt would jockey from the kitchen to the dining room to periodically check on my uncle and would make the same comment year after year,"*No matter what I make, you have nothing good to say, and why don't you use the saucer next to your plate to put all that stuff in, instead of putting it all over my table?*" My uncle would either ignore her or simply feign deafness. Later on, I realized that this was simply their way of garnering each other's attention. It was their little ritual, and all of their petty jests and jibes were the norm, leaving us all to chuckle and wonder. When all was said and done, and aside from all the playful ribbing, it was abundantly clear that the two of them were deeply in love.

My uncle and I had a special bond that extended from the warm place in his heart that he reserved for my mother. My mother's mother was debilitated by what I now believe to have been a stubborn case of resistance to authority. Combined with postpartum depression, my grandmother became infirm in her later years. My grandfather mostly coped by disengaging from everyday life and working alone outdoors much of the time. This left his youngest child, my mother, largely to her own devices, and it was ultimately my uncle who took on the responsibility of raising her. My birth added to his instinctive desire to nurture and a lifelong kinship ensued.

When I arrived in his house during my summer holidays from Northern India, my uncle would show off to his own children how he and I could speak in English, while the cousins stood by, displaying a mixture of admiration and resentment. There were times when I would burn with embarrassment, feeling unworthy of an affection that my uncle withheld from his own offspring, but uncle would persist, and our relationship became and remained strong.

Often, after dinner, my uncle would disappear into his study, reappearing moments later with a tall, oval tin of extra fancy Cadbury chocolates. He would put two of them in my palm, smiling as if it was our little secret. My mother told me that, when I was a premature, frail infant, and her milk was insufficient in nourishing me, that my uncle, unbeknownst to my aunt, ordered expensive baby formula regularly and gave it to my mother. My uncle and I have a very special bond.

Aunt Lily spent most of her days mulling around the kitchen, preparing meals for the family. Unquestionably, her dishes exuded exceptional elegance and zest. Maybe it was because she could afford to use more coconut oil or that she managed to acquire higher quality ingredients, carefully guarded in her cupboard. But even more than this, she was a magician of sorts, able to take simple ingredients and give them that extra, special touch. Her appams, egg curries, vegetable sautés and lentils were all superb! My favorite dish of all, though, was one that was of lowly origin, favored by laborers and landlords alike: her Sautéed Brown Beans.

Sautéed Brown Beans
Vanpayar Olarthiade

Vanpayar is also known as brown peas, cow peas, or Chinese string beans. In its raw, green bean form known as *Payar,* it is one of Kerala's favorite vegetables. Its nut-like, savory flavor makes it taste much richer and more satisfying than the common green bean. Whether it is sautéed with onion and pieces of coconut, or finely chopped and cooked with grated coconut, it is a dish everyone loves.

Vanpayar is made from the dried kernels of the ripe beans. After soaking them for a few hours in water, they can then be boiled and made into various dishes, including sautés, curries and mashes. Loaded with protein and fiber, this bean dish is considered the poor man's meat in Kerala, and with the help of Aunt Lily's culinary wizardry, each mouthful turned into an aromatic explosion of flavors.

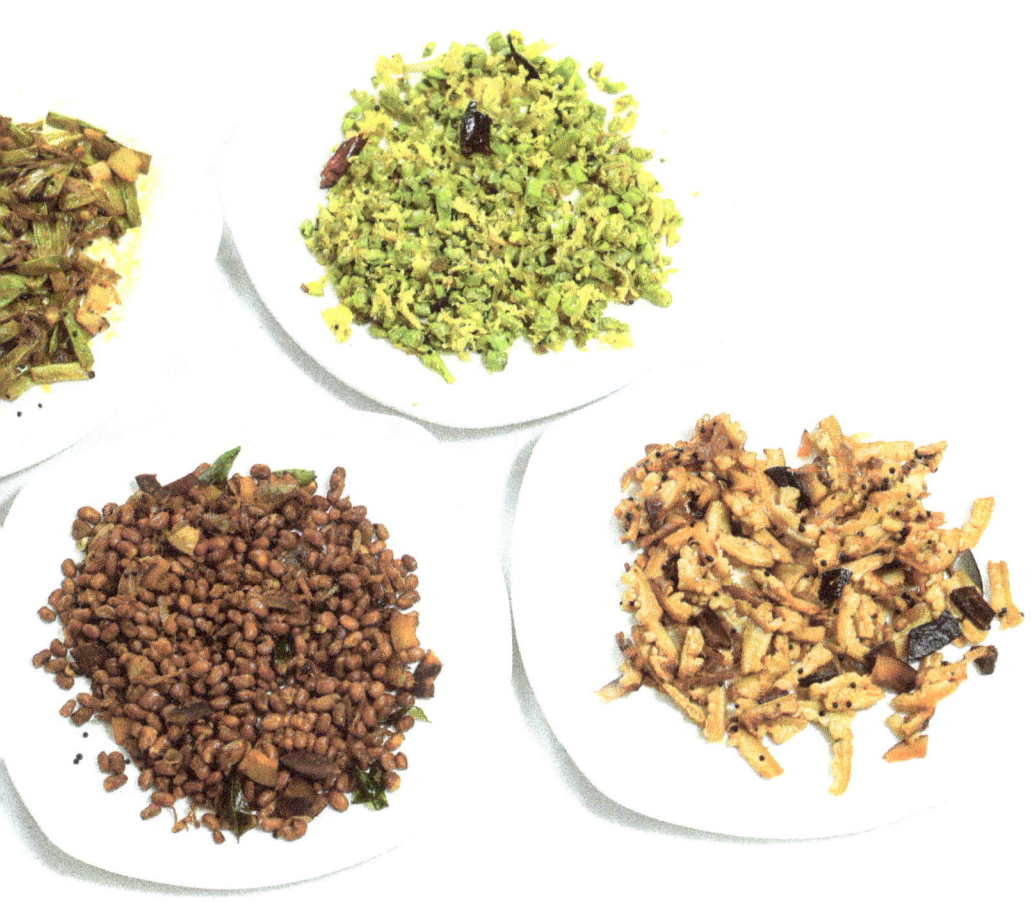

Aunt Lily's Sautéed Brown Beans
Vanpayar Olarthiade

Ingredients

2 cups brown beans (available in Indian stores and some organic grocery stores. These are brown versions of black-eyed-peas)

½ medium sized red onion

2 dried red chilis roughly crushed (or just broken in half if you cannot tolerate spicy heat)

10 – 15 fresh curry leaves

2 tbsp coconut oil

Salt to taste

Process

- Soak beans overnight, or for 6-8 hours
- Boil in six cups of water until beans cooked to desired consistency. The beans can remain somewhat firm but cooked, medium or even overcooked, depending on individual preference.
- Drain beans and leave in cauldron until ready.
- Roughly crush onion and dried chili in a mortar and keep aside.
- Heat the coconut oil in a deep frying pan or wok *(Be careful not to burn the oil)*.
- Add crushed onion and red chili and curry leaves, turn heat to desired level so that ingredients do not burn. Stir constantly.
- Add beans and salt to taste and increase heat. Stir constantly until the nutty aroma of the beans fills the kitchen.

Serve with rice, flatbreads, breads, quinoa or tapioca (traditionally served with rice and spiced buttermilk.).

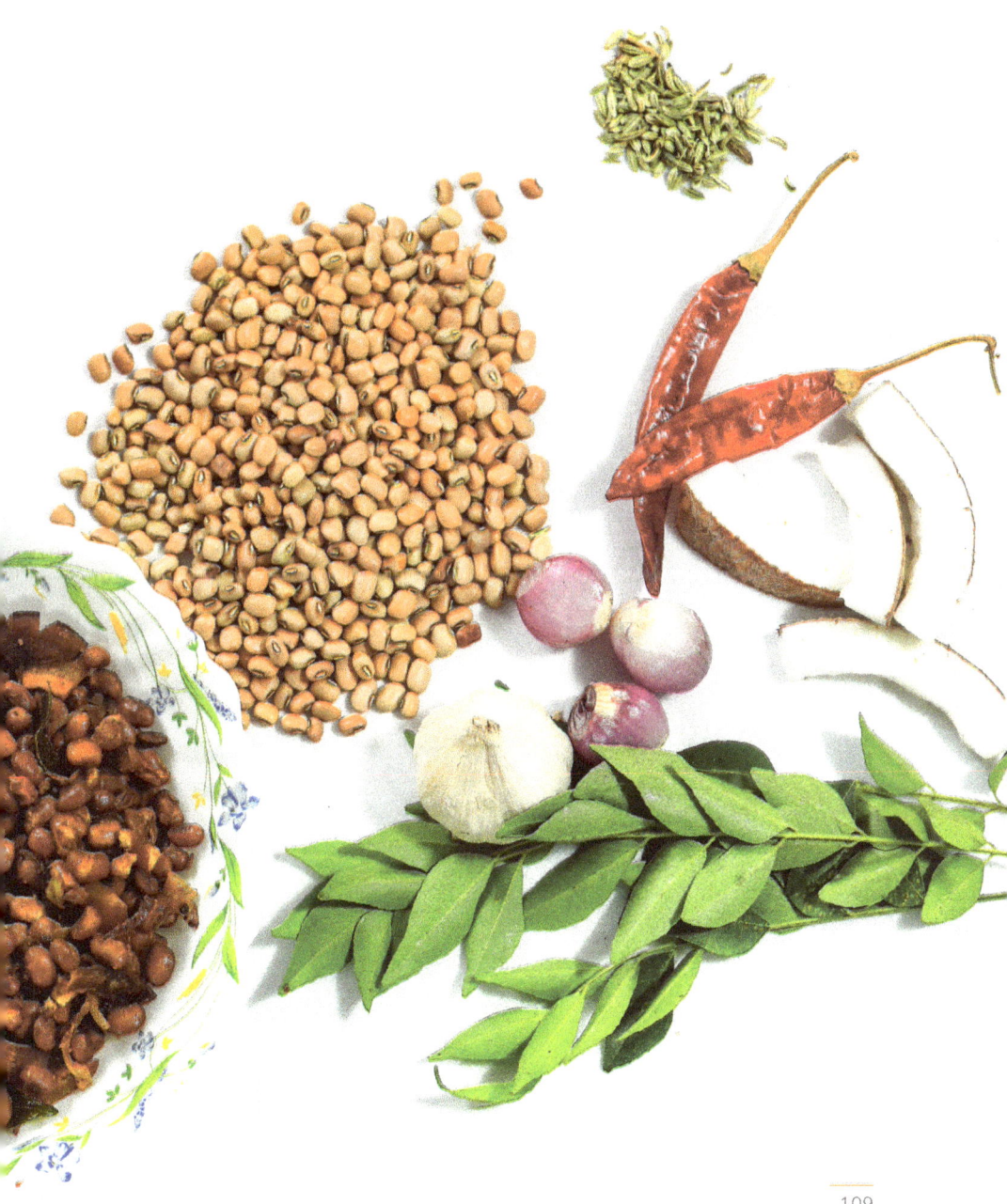

SPICED MASHED POTATOES
Kizangu Masala

Though small quantities of potatoes appear in many Keralan recipes, there are only a few in which potatoes are the prominent ingredient. One of these is the *masala* that is used as stuffing in the famous **Masala Dosa**. **Dosa** is a paper thin, crispy crepe made from rice and lentils. Potatoes requiring cooler climates arrive in Kerala from the high ranges of northern Kerala, neighboring states, and northern India. Potatoes were brought to India by the Portuguese on the west coast, and by the British to Calcutta in the east.

I do not remember **Masala Dosa** being made when I visited Kerala in my youth. I do, however, recall that I was first introduced to **Masala Dosa** during one of my journeys through Changanacherry, the town that lay roughly halfway between my paternal and maternal ancestral homes. A stop in Changanacherry was common, either to have **Appam** and Egg Roast at an eating hall at the boat jetty, or **Masala Dosa** at the only vegetarian restaurant in town. The **Masala Dosa** did not make an impression on me until a few years later, when I was nearly nine years old, and my uncle took me to the *Indian Coffee House*.

The *Indian Coffee House*s were first introduced to India by the British in 1937, when approximately forty outlets sprung up throughout the country in an effort to promote coffee drinking and the sale of coffee beans. These outlets, however, were closed down in 1940 due to lack of patronage. The concept was resurrected in 1957 as a cooperative movement, co-owned and operated by its own employees, a practice which continues to this very day.

These coffee houses were meeting places for students and professionals, and even, on occasion, a destination for families with children. These upscale watering holes were the only places during my childhood and adolescent years in India where the quality of the product was excellent and predictable. The exceptional coffees and teas satisfied the palate each and every visit, without fail, and the snacks served were of noteworthy quality. In addition to beverages, these eateries also served mostly South Indian **Masala Dosa, Idli, Uzhunnu Vada, samosas,** and a few other indigenous staples.

Entering an establishment of this type was also very different in another rare and exclusive way: the attention of young and old alike were drawn to the ornate, Maharaja-style capes that the servers donned, replete with a white pleated fan that spread outward, upon opening, in proud, peacock style. The servers' white uniforms also stood out in contrast to their red, embroidered insignia on the front, reminding one of the imperial days, and perhaps in deference to how the "rulers" were once approached. The whole atmosphere was a bit surreal yet inestimably inviting, and, at least for the time we were there, we felt as if we were being treated like royalty!

The children particularly fancied the pageantry of the place, especially when a server emerged majestically, wielding a white plate held up on his palm with the almost two feet long **Masala Dosa** *sticking* out on either side of the plate like a bird's wings. We watched expectantly as the server placed the food, in high fashion and with a flourish, on the table, his serious demeanor never giving way to a hint of levity. We were awed.

As soon as the food was brought out, we began eagerly breaking off crispy edges of the ***dosa*** and jabbing it into the stuffed midsection of the dish, so as to pinch up the yellow ***potato masala*** (now also available in red color with beetroot juice added). We washed it down with a magnificent sip of tea or coffee.

Over the years I have noticed that, both in Kerala and in Jabalpur (in northern India where I grew up), ***potato masala*** was a favorite dish to pair with ***chapati, puri, paratha,*** or other Indian flatbreads.

I visited an Indian coffeehouse during my last visit in 2018 to Kerala. The place was full and bustling, the location perfect, and the food was quite good. The building, which seemed like a very old British bungalow, looked run down and in need of a lot of repair. Except fo r the Maître D', who wore the full uniform and ornate headgear, none of the servers were outfitted as in the past. The place was more reminiscent of a cafeteria, lacking its original formality and grandeur. The Golden Jubilee of the Indian Coffee House occurred in 2018, and there are efforts that are now underway to revamp it, hopefully returning it to the magic of its former years.

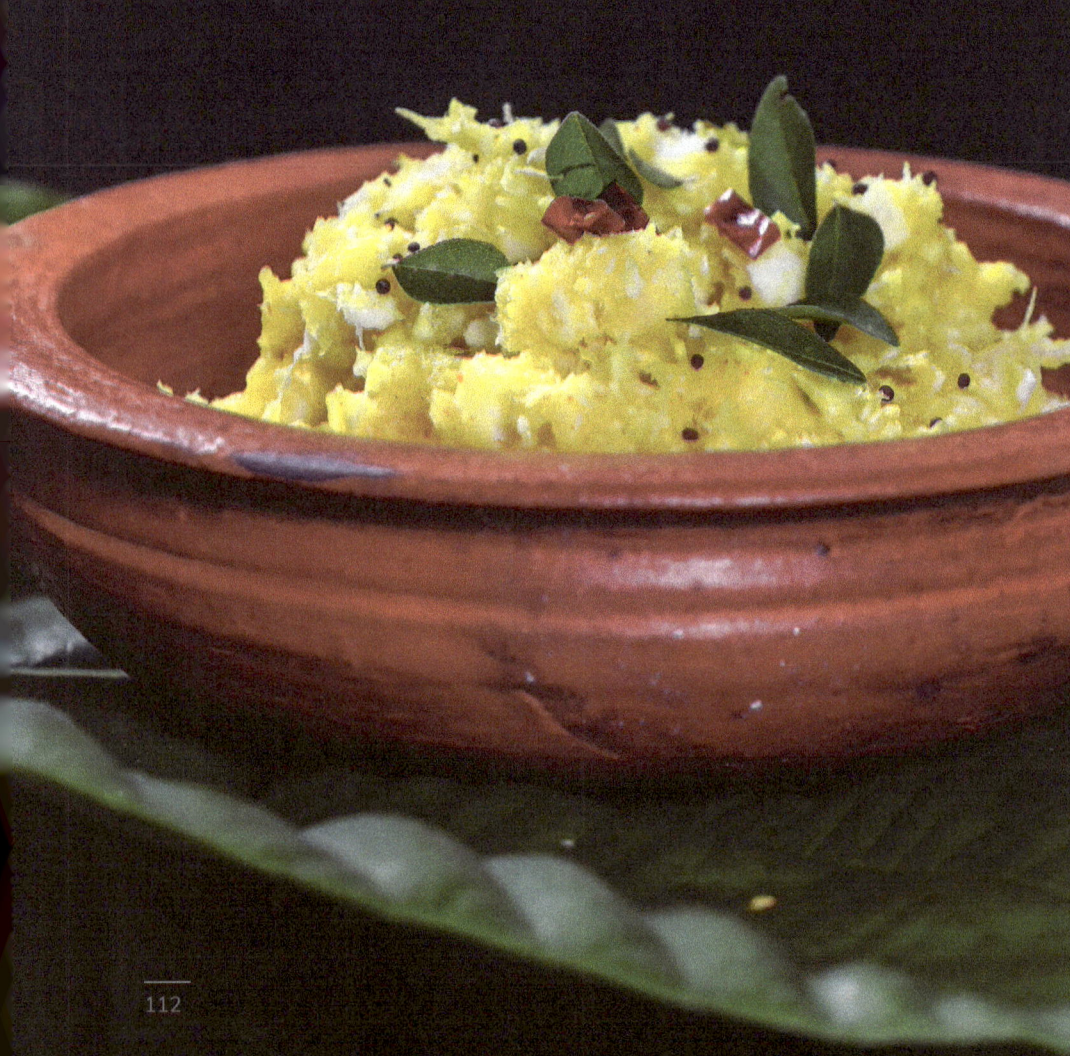

Spiced Mashed Potatoes
Kizangu Masala

Ingredients

5-6 medium sized potatoes (1lb)

½ medium sized white onion roughly chopped

1 green chili, whole

3-4 cloves garlic, sliced lengthwise

½ inch fresh ginger, peeled and crushed roughly

½ cup of roughly chopped cilantro, or 10-14 fresh curry leaves if available

½ tsp mustard seeds

½ tsp cumin seeds

¼ tsp turmeric

3-4 dashes of asafetida

2 dried red chilies; leave whole, or break in half if able to tolerate spicy heat

1 tbsp oil of choice

Process

- Peel, boil and mash potatoes to a rough consistency, with small chunks of potatoes still remaining in the mixture.
- Heat oil in a deep pan or wok.
- Place mustard and cumin seeds and dried red chilies in the oil. Cover lightly with gap until mustard seeds pop. Then add in the asafetida.
- Turn heat down to medium and add onions, ginger and garlic, green chili (and curry leaves if used).
- Sauté on medium heat, stirring often until onions caramelize
- Lower heat and add turmeric and chili powder.
- Stir for 1 minute.
- Add mashed potatoes and salt to taste and mix ingredients thoroughly.
- Pat down and cover with a tight lid. Turn off heat.

*Serve with any flatbread, tortillas, **nans**, in a sandwich, or stuffed in a **dosa**.*

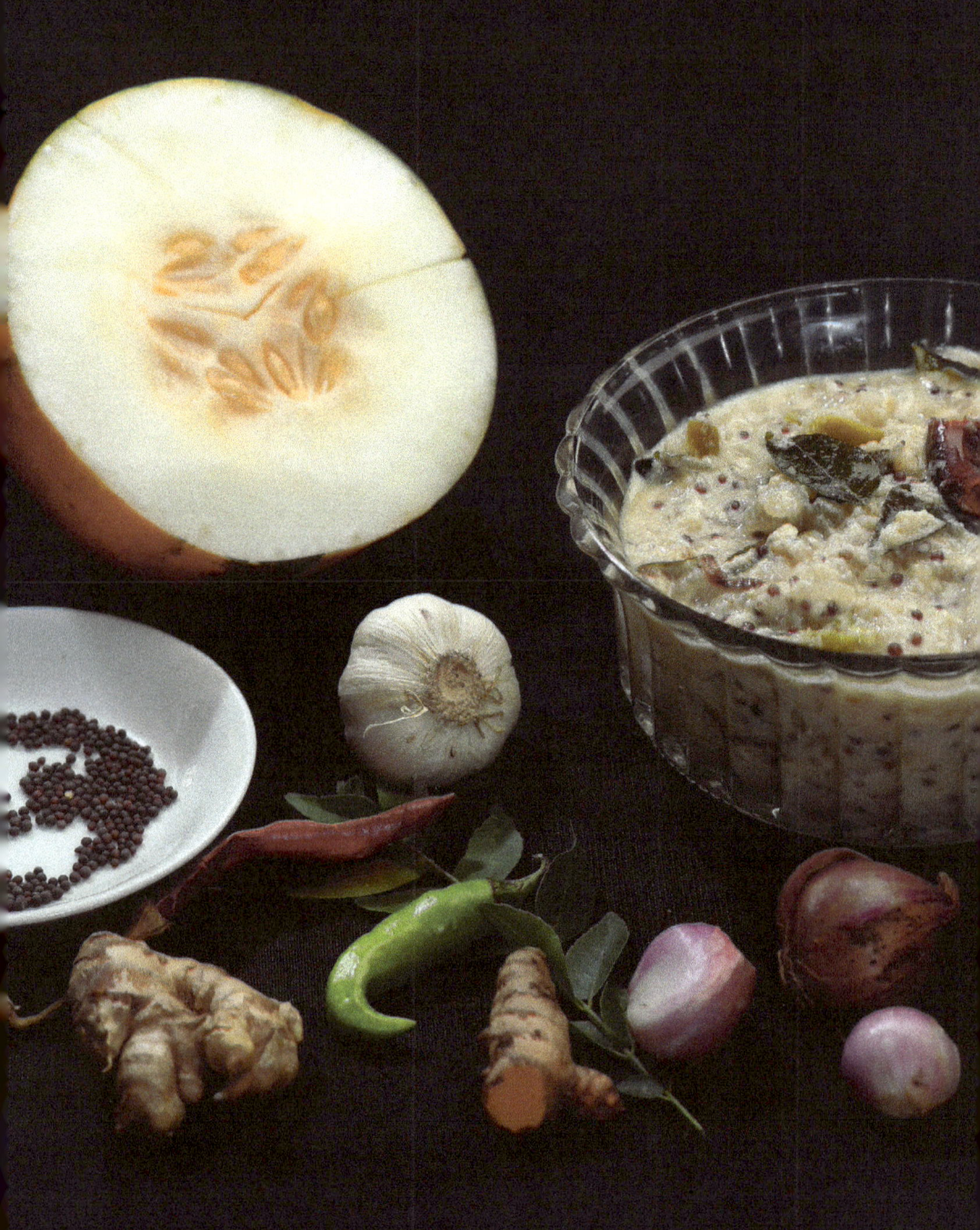

Yogurt Pacchadi

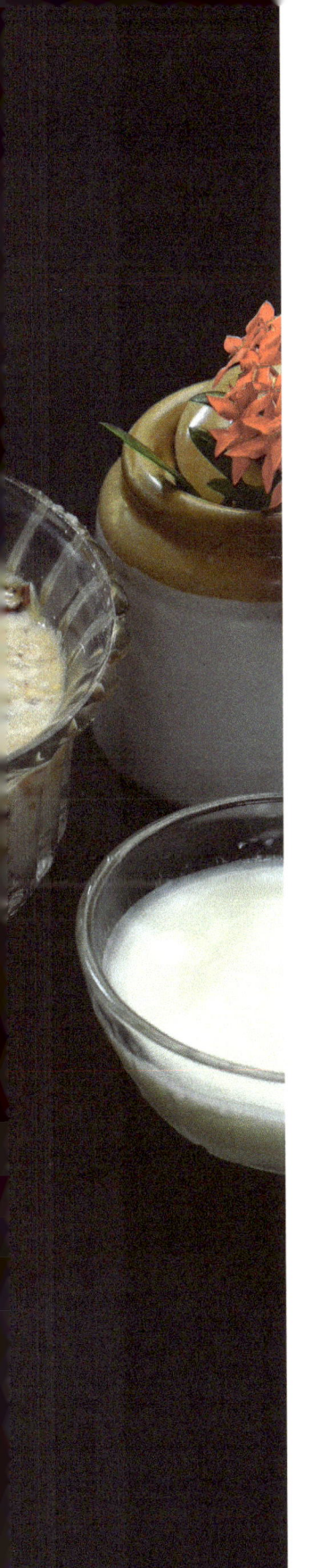

YOGURT DISHES

GOLDEN SPICED BUTTERMILK
Kachimore

Grandma's kitchen was one of the biggest rooms in the house, located on the far end, with a separate entrance for daily harvest deliveries from the surrounding land. On most days, Grandma or one the aunts would step out into the lush, wild foliage and reap whatever was ready to be eaten: **payar** (Chinese string beans), okra, **cheera** (crimson or green Kerala spinach), **pavakka** (bitter gourd), **padavalanga** (snake gourd) and many other excellent and exotic varieties of edible plants. Sometimes this activity involved shaking or pulling down raw mangoes, drumsticks (Moringa pods), papayas or other fruits from tall trees. At other times, the yield consisted of gorgeous turmeric or finger-like ginger if and when fresh roots were needed.

The remainder of the ingredients, such as dry spices, grains and other staples, were gathered from the room adjacent to the kitchen. This room, in addition to serving as Grandma's bedroom with her tiny cot near the window, was also a *de facto* storage room. Turmeric, ginger root, black pepper, rice tied neatly in gunny sacks, cardamom, cloves, cinnamon sticks wrapped in delicate cloth bundles, nutmeg and other

From the beginning of recorded history, human beings have sought out this Malabar Coast, looking for spices. This includes the descendants of Abraham, the Ancient Romans, Chinese, British, Dutch, Arabs, and the Italian adventurer Christopher Columbus. Today, these same seasonings have found their way to the hearths and hearts of the New World, offering flavors that have the ability to both delight and heal.

condiments were stacked on the floor on the other end of the room, away from the window where exposure to light could damage their potency. Here, in this quiet, private space, Grandma preferred to both sleep and work her culinary magic.

In Grandma's kitchen, suspended from the timber supports of the shelf over the hearth, porcelain or clay pots held various cooking staples, including rock salt, fermenting yogurt, spiced buttermilk **Kachimoru** and tamarind, to name a few. Many other staples like seasonal fish and pickled vegetables or fruits were strategically placed in different corners behind the hearth so that the smoke and heat preserved them and infused them with aromatic flavors.

Kanji (rice porridge), rendered golden yellow with **Kachimoru**, a buttermilk dish flavored with roasted fenugreek, cumin, turmeric and a half dozen other common spices, is what Grandma served if any of the children had the mildest stomach upset. Served warm, in large, white, deep-bellied saucers called **Coopas,** it was the tastiest potion imaginable and one that would put any tummy back on solid ground.

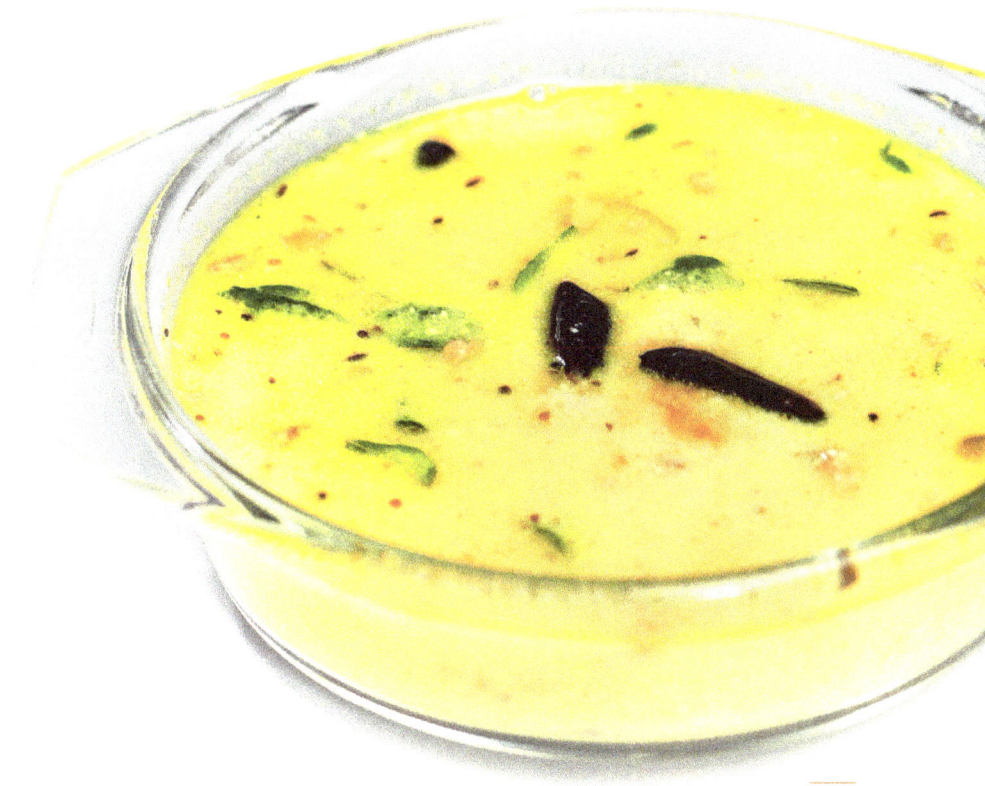

Golden Spiced Buttermilk
Kachimoru

Ingredients

- 8 oz whole milk yogurt
- 6 oz room temperature water
- 1 tbsp coconut oil
- 1 dried red chili broken into 2-3 pieces
- 2 tbsp finely chopped onions or shallots
- 1 green chili with stem, whole, sliced in the middle without separating
- 2 tsp finely chopped or crushed ginger root
- 2 tsp turmeric powder
- 1-3 medium sized cloves of garlic roughly chopped
- 1 tsp fenugreek seeds
- ½ tsp mustard seeds
- ½ tsp cumin seeds
- 2-3 dashes of Asafetida
- ½ tsp whole black peppercorns
- Fresh or dried curry leaves whole, 10-15 leaves (can substitute fresh cilantro leaves roughly chopped, if curry leaves are not available)
- Sea salt to taste

Process

- Blend water and yogurt with whisk (or lightly in blender) for seconds until milky consistency.
- Heat stainless steel, medium sized cooking pan.
- Place coconut oil in the pan on medium to low heat.
- Add fenugreek, cumin, mustard, dried chili, peppercorns and curry leaves to the hot oil (do not let oil burn).
- Cover lightly with mesh or the lid, leaving a small opening.
- When mustard seeds pop, add 2-3 dashes of Asafetida.
- Add onion, green chili, ginger, garlic, then sauté (add cilantro if using instead of curry leaves) until browned.
- Lower heat and add turmeric powder.
- Cook the remaining time on very low heat with constant stirring until the mixture is medium hot to the touch of a finger but not very hot or boiling.
- Continue stirring the mixture on low heat for another 5 minutes.
- Cool the mixture.
- Pour the mixture into a glass or porcelain container.

Serve over rice; can also be eaten as a soup.

It can be stored in the refrigerator for 3-5 days or until the mixture tastes too sour. It can also be left at room temperature in winter or cold climates.

Grandma's Kitchen Staple, served frequently with rice.

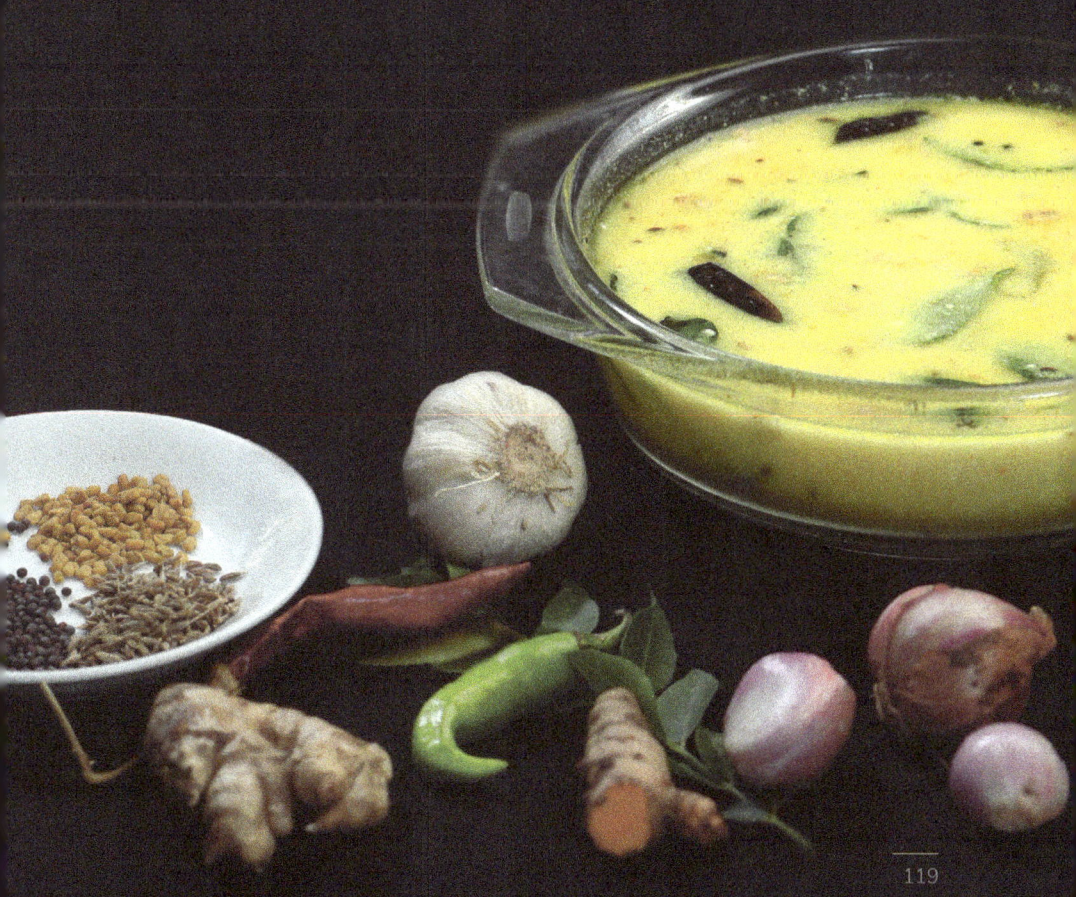

MALI'S KONKANI YOGURT RICE

Malini, my mother-in-law, affectionately called Mali by her peers and "Amma" by me and the generations that followed her, came into my life in 1978. At first, I only knew her from a distance, gathering bits and pieces about her from what my husband told me and from conversations I heard when he called home on Saturdays. Phone calls were unaffordable, and the minutes had to be counted. An exchange about Amma's most recent cooking was critical, no matter how short the conversation was. My husband sorely missed his mother's culinary expertise. He seemed to derive vicarious pleasure from these discussions.

Amma could not be present for our American court wedding in 1978. She attended our church wedding, which took place two years later, at the Jesu Chapel of Marquette University. My parents were devout Catholics and needed a Catholic wedding to legitimize the bond, but it took them two years to save up the funds to attend the event. It would also take us six months of CANA, Catholic premarital counseling, every Friday when Father Simon would come to our home to counsel us and enjoy my version of rice, beef curry, and spinach **Raita**.

My husband and I both arrived in the United States in 1978. He was 21, working on his master's degree at Marquette University. I emigrated at 18 with my family to live in America. I enrolled at Marquette University in the fall of 1978 as an undergraduate.

We were from different parts of India. Culturally, we were worlds apart, but through our common education in India, we understood and related to the modernity and culture of the Western world. Communication between us was somewhat natural and effortless.

In addition to studying science, math, history and geography, I had grown up on a diet consisting of Mark Twain, Thomas Mann, Tolstoy and Tagore. Grand landscapes depicted by James Michener gave me glimpses of the Chesapeake Bay, as well as other treasures of the New World. I dreamed about the places I had visited in books, hoping that I would, one day, have the opportunity to actually live in them.

I did not hear much about my husband's literary interests when he was growing up. It was clear that cricket and judo consumed his attention and that he was a frequent visitor to the American Embassy, determined to leave India in search of a better life. Moreover, he apparently had memorized the curricula and educational prospecti of many American universities.

While still a high school student, my future husband had indulged in a few coming-of-age adventures, taken straight from the pages of a Harold Robbins novel that had circulated amongst his classmates and which we laughed about later. Fortunately, he continued to mature, and during his early educational tenure, a transatlantic letter-writing friendship developed between him and a professor at Marquette University, ultimately procuring him place in the master's program there. His passage from India was a success.

For both of us, English was our first language, and we could communicate in Hindi as well, the national language of India. Over the ensuing years, we picked up quite a bit of each other's vernaculars. I learned some *Konkani* (the language of his ancestors from Konkan) and *Marathi* (the language of the state of Maharashtra, and city of Mumbai, where he was born and raised) while my husband acquired enough *Malayalam* (the language of Kerala where I was born) for both of us to understand gossip and fun as well as completely and hilariously misunderstand more serious issues when we met with each other's families.

My husband was born and raised in the famous city of Bombay, now renamed *Mumbai*, on the western coast of India. I was born in Kerala and was raised in the sleepy army town of Jabalpur in the heart of India, in the state of *Madhya Pradesh*, which literally translates to "the state in the middle of India." I was raised a traditional Catholic, deeply entrenched in its religious dogma and tradition, with both my parents' families producing priests, bishops and nuns.

From the age of nine, I grew up attending daily Mass and was raised with the mantra of frugality, service and guilt. Overindulgence in anything, whether it was clothing, personal luxury, or food left my conscience bruised and produced anxiety and repentance. I grew up eating everything but enjoyed non-vegetarian dishes only on occasion. On weekdays, the fare leaned more to the lighter side, and, on Saturdays and Sundays, meat or fish would be served. Everything was measured and sparse.

My husband, on the other hand, was raised in a non-traditional, Konkani Brahmin family. His ancestors migrated from Konkan in the state then known as Mysore, from towns like Udupi and Dharwad, that are considered to embody the heart of Hinduism. There the highest caste of Brahmins are trained in *Maths,* which are monasteries that still exist today. In these *Maths,* and beginning at a young age, boys from Hindu Brahmin families were groomed to become temple priests, sacred mortals who held the secrets of the language and power of Hindu rituals. These chosen ones were trained in the philosophy, rites and traditions of this religious discipline. My husband's family had nothing to do with any of this, except for his initiation ceremony called the "the thread ceremony," or the ritualistic donning of the "holy thread" across the torso that designates the symbolic rite of passage from boyhood into the adult responsibilities of a Brahmin.

My husband's father had worked in the Airport customs department. He had many Christian friends so the cuisine in his household developed into two disparate categories: one extremely traditional ***sattvic*** (spirituality-enhancing), pure vegetarian, Konkani Brahmin cooking, and the other a blasphemously non-vegetarian, rich, ***rajasic/tamasic*** (stimulating) style, including all manner of flesh—beef, pork, mutton and sausages—introduced to my father-in-law by his well-meaning, Christian friends. Throughout his young life, my husband's home became a hub for non-vegetarian cuisine, for extended members of his family and for Hindu friends who wanted to indulge in that which was considered taboo, unbeknownst to their families.

Amma, a free spirit, loved cooking and serving and enjoyed her craft no matter what was served. Her world revolved around the meals and get-togethers in her tiny two room flat in Mumbai, a valuable piece of real estate bequeathed to her by her wealthy businessman father. Her mother was a pure vegetarian and did not eat either fish or meat.

The original Konkani Brahmin recipes, handed over to Mali by her mother and aunts, were protected and followed in every detail, without deviating or adding her own touches to the original formula. These dishes were simple, easy to make, and left one with a sense of pure satisfaction.

As with other immigrants, a significant number of Brahmins leave the country to become professionals in the developed world, gravitating especially to the United States. Most quickly shed any semblance of this culture in order to integrate seamlessly into the New World. The old customs and rituals were often discarded as superstitious and archaic.

Dahi Bhat, which means "yogurt rice," is one of these recipes that again could fall into the category of "Food of the Gods." The simple recipe produces a burst of tastes and flavors that are easy on the palate, and providing excellent, comforting, and affordable nutrition for the rich and poor alike. On hot summer days, a meal of only **Dahi Bhat** by itself, leaves one cool, satisfied and cleansed.

My adult children still ask me to make this dish to remember their childhood with Amma, who came every other year for decades to be with us. Amma played an integral role in raising them, moving here permanently in later years, in order to be with her family, visit with other members of the tribe, and catch up with her soap operas, which were not available in the East.

Konkani yogurt rice is the dish that my own children, decades later, still yearn for to purge themselves when they are fed up with burgers, pizzas, fried chicken, BBQ and fancy meals at expensive restaurants.

Amma's Konkani Yogurt Rice
Dahi Bath

Ingredients

2 cups basmati rice

1-1.5 cups organic whole milk yogurt

1 tsp mustard seed

1 tsp cumin

½ tsp black peppercorns

1-2 green chili (left whole sliced partially lengthwise without separating the two slices. This can be left out if one cannot tolerate spicy heat)

1-2 dried red chili whole

10-15 fresh curry leaves (one can substitute fresh cilantro if curry leaves not available)

1 tsp finely chopped white onion 1tsp finely crushed fresh ginger root

Asafetida

1 tbsp coconut oil, olive oil, or other vegetable oil of choice

Salt to taste

Process

- Wash Basmati rice thoroughly in cold water and drain.
- Add 4.5 cups of water and cook initially on high heat, uncovered, until boiling, then cover and lower heat to lowest level, until rice is thoroughly cooked (even slightly overcooked is okay), and set aside.
- In a larger, stainless dish, mix rice and yogurt (1-1.5 cups based on desired consistency; one can add more or less yogurt), and salt to taste. Crush wiith clean hand until thoroughly mixed and rice grains are slightly crushed. Set aside.
- In sauce pan or wok, heat oil and add mustard seeds, cumin seeds, peppercorns, dried red chili, and half of the curry leaves, then lower heat to medium and cover lightly with gap until mustard pops (If using cilantro instead of curry leaves do NOT add any cilantro at this stage).
- Add onions, ginger, green chili, the remaining curry leaves, 1-3 dashes of asafetida. Increase heat to high and stir for a minute until contents turn dark brown.
- Pour contents of sauce pan immediately over the prepared rice.

If using fresh cilantro instead of curry leaves, add fresh chopped cilantro at the end of cooking and mix contents thoroughly with a wooden spoon.

*Serve at room temperature or cooled in fridge on hot summer days with Indian **achar**. South Asian pickles or achar are pickled foods, native to India, made from a variety of vegetables and fruits, preserved in brine, vinegar, or oils along with spices.*

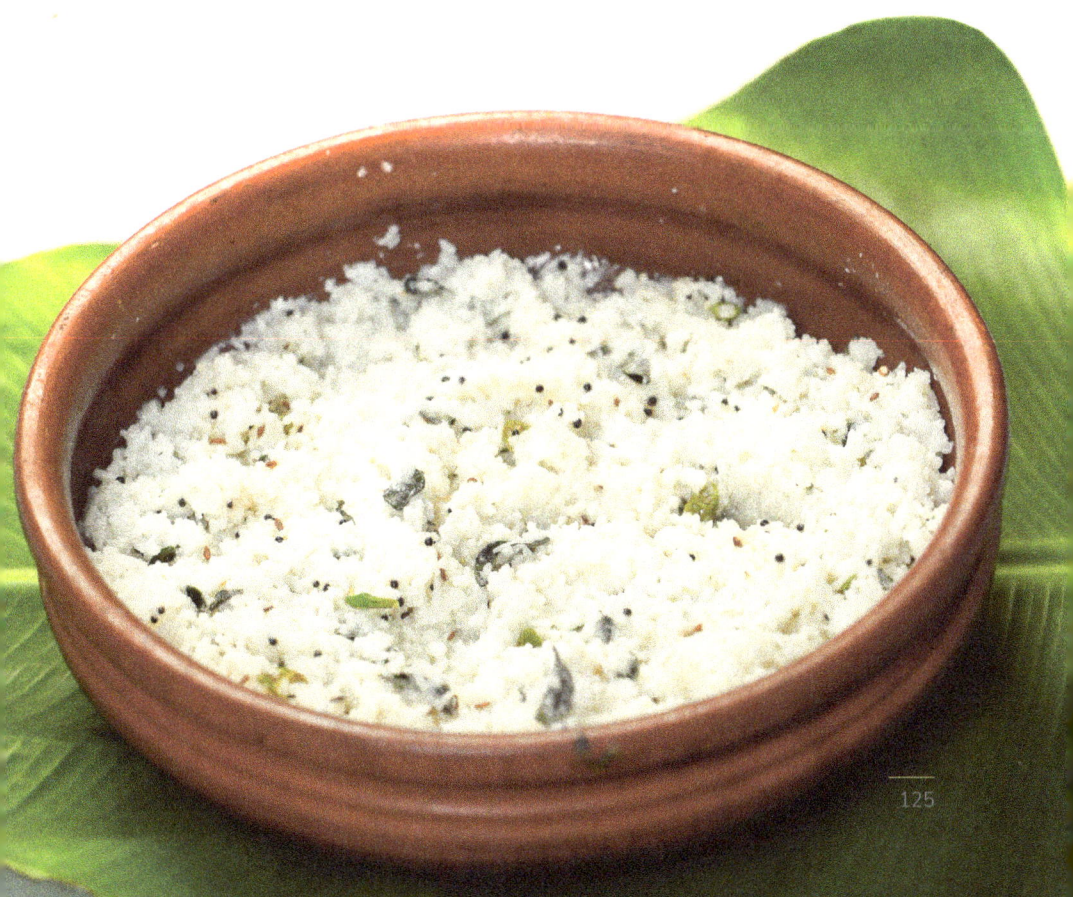

MALI AND MIRIAM'S YOGURT DISHES
Pacchadi and Raita

Growing up, I was exposed to Keralan and other native versions of yogurt dishes from northern India. Each one had a distinctly different method of preparation, as well as an easily distinguishable and unique taste. Raw yogurt dishes seemed to predominate in the north, while Keralan and other southern versions leaned heavily toward the cooked variety.

Common to both locales was the milk, which came from cows that belonged to the family or their neighbors, and yogurt was almost always made at home. Each time that a cow gave birth to a baby calf, we children would stand nearby, watching with great curiosity as the calf first stood unsteadily on its new-found legs. Then a calf opened its eyes wide trying mightily to steady its gaze from its head perched on its still unstable neck. We marveled at how this fragile creature gravitated instantly towards its mother's udders. We were absolutely mesmerized by the gentleness and love with which the mother licked her calf until its coat was dry and shiny, and it was ready to face the world.

In the days to follow, each one of us would take our turn making friends with the calf, naming it, stroking its forehead, and making eye contact. This patient interaction culminated a day or two later in a cuddly, amiable hug. Those were the days when we would rush home from school, racing to be the first to reach the barn, to bask in the wonder of our family's new arrival. We would rarely come empty-handed, every banana peel, each bit of fruit or clump of tender grass, would be rushed to the baby and mother, then hand-fed to them as a morsel of love and gratitude. This was our friendship ritual and the forming of a bond that would last for years.

At the appropriate juncture, the calf would be tied up close to the mother, fettered to her using a length of rope that was just long enough to keep the baby away from her mother's swollen udders. Finally, the day would come, and the baby would have to share her mother's delicious milk with us! This milk would arrive in our kitchen in steel buckets, warm and frothy with a saccharine, baby-like scent that sent one's taste buds dancing. Even though milk was such a precious commodity even back then, for a few weeks at least, we were permitted to drink liberally from our cow's prized offering. We sipped it hot, spiked with turmeric and sugar at bedtime and we blended it into our *chai* twice a day. Yogurt and *ghee* would also become more abundant for a few months, by-products of this same gift. Finally, some of the milk would be sold to the neighbors to supplement the family income.

Central to Grandma's home and hearth was the designated, red clay pot. This esteemed vessel, used over and over again in the making of so many favorite dishes and treats, had turned black from the soot bestowed on it from the wood-fired stove. Every evening, Grandma, or one of the aunts, took on the task of boiling and cooling the milk until it was lukewarm then mixed into it a scoop of the previous day's yogurt. The warmth of the hearth, combined with the primordial bacteria in the yogurt culture would then work their magic, fermenting the mixture overnight, and transforming it from a buttery, silky milk into a pleasantly sweet and sour, sumptuous jelly-like yogurt. In the meanwhile, the bacteria intrinsic to this process had multiplied a thousand fold, in preparation for the new home these microscopic creatures would find upon entry into the human gut.

Modern medical science has discovered that the number of these bacteria, now called probiotics or gut biome, exceed the number of cells in our bodies by a hundredfold or more. The lining of each segment of our twenty two feet of gut can be thought of as different countries, inhabited by unique populations of these helpful bacteria. These trillions of organisms literally and figuratively make up yet another complex living organism, similar to the billions of cells in our body that co-exist and that make us human. Together, and in symbiotic fashion, they work in tandem to bring about a measure of gut health that is simply unavailable otherwise. With them, we are truly a "super-organism;" without, a being that bows to the mercy of the elements.

Scientists and philosophers are asking the question as to who qualifies as the host in this partnership: are we secondary to the gut biome or does the gut biome cling to us? It is now being discovered that this living "Nano-carpet" lining our gut is the gatekeeper, determining what does and does not enter our innards. Moreover, it also micro-manages how things enter, knowing with an intelligence we can barely fathom, what is required by the body and what should be excluded.

As an example, we are discovering that the proportions and types of these bacteria are linked to how carbohydrates, fats and proteins are absorbed into our body. We are also getting more insight into the effect that fasting, overconsumption, antibiotics, hormones and processed foods affect the relative and absolute number of these bacteria that can survive in our inner environment. Many critical micronutrients and vitamins, such as vitamin K, folate, thiamine, riboflavin, and other water-soluble vitamins, require the help of gut bacteria for their proper absorption.

Researchers are now making more and greater discoveries, linking the gut biome to the health of our immune system. We are, like never before, privy to scientific insights into the ways in which many diseases, from cancer to autoimmune diseases, autism and even many mental illnesses, may be inextricably linked to the health or altered states of these crucial gut bacteria.

By virtue of centuries of experience, our forefathers seemed to have acquired many valuable lessons from nature, and even without being able to explain the mechanistic nature of the processes, they were able to observe and humbly take a lesson from these cognitions, imbibing and following the teachings of the plants and animals in their lives.

Yes, the cow was worshipped! After all, it provided complex sustenance, milk to grow us from infancy to adults, butter, yogurt, food for our other partner the gut biome, manure to grow the plants that sustained us, and provided us clothing and shelter. Perhaps most all, this animal teaches us lessons in selfless love and tolerance.

Today, the industrial revolution has taught us to short circuit this gentle journey of caring and mutual nurturing. We have opted to go for the jugular—to the dead body of the animal after the spirit has left. The caustic impact of factory-farmed, polluted and poisonous meats, ingested day after day, as our primary source of nutrition, has left us with heart disease, and not just the physical kind, composed of clogs and blockages, but also the spiritual type. We suffer from broken hearts starving for connection and companionship. Factory farming has converted "cows" to "livestock," donning them with numbers that secure their position on the "cash cow" scale, and the slaughter queue. Today, we can acquire parts of these beasts in neat little packets, sold in massive bulk at behemoth super stores, whenever, wherever and however we please. If this ends up being too much effort, we can even purchase them in "ready to be consumed" quantities, effortlessly deposited in our waiting laps, never having to leave the luxury of our heated or cooled vehicles, as we enter and exit the drive-thru window of the fast food joint, arched or otherwise.

Ironically, medical science is coming full circle as we speak. Humans are slowly but surely realizing the monstrous error of their ways, and are, instead, gravitating toward the gentle, the organic, the meager and the mindful. They are revisiting the notion, that cows and calves can occupy a place, not only on our dining tables, but in our hearts and souls, and that real yogurt and butter can ferment on our very own kitchen counters, producing genuine, wholesome, healing food that is nourishing and delicious. This book is a testimony to that effort.

Mali's Cucumber or Spinach Raita

Ingredients

2 cup organic plain whole milk yogurt

1 large cucumber peeled and grated; cucumber can be replaced with zucchini, or cooked, chopped spinach (frozen organic spinach, thawed and cooked for 3-5 min, covered, works best)

1 tsp of fresh ginger, crushed or finely grated

¼ of medium-sized red onion, diced into fine cubes

¼ tsp ground pepper

Asafetida 2-3 dashes

Salt to taste

½ cup fresh cilantro chopped (skip cilantro if making Spinach **Raita**)

Finely powdered Himalayan salt if available, 1-2 pinches

Process

- Mix ingredients 1-7 in a serving dish
- Garnish with cilantro for cucumber **Raita**
- Also garnish with 1-2 pinches of Himalayan salt

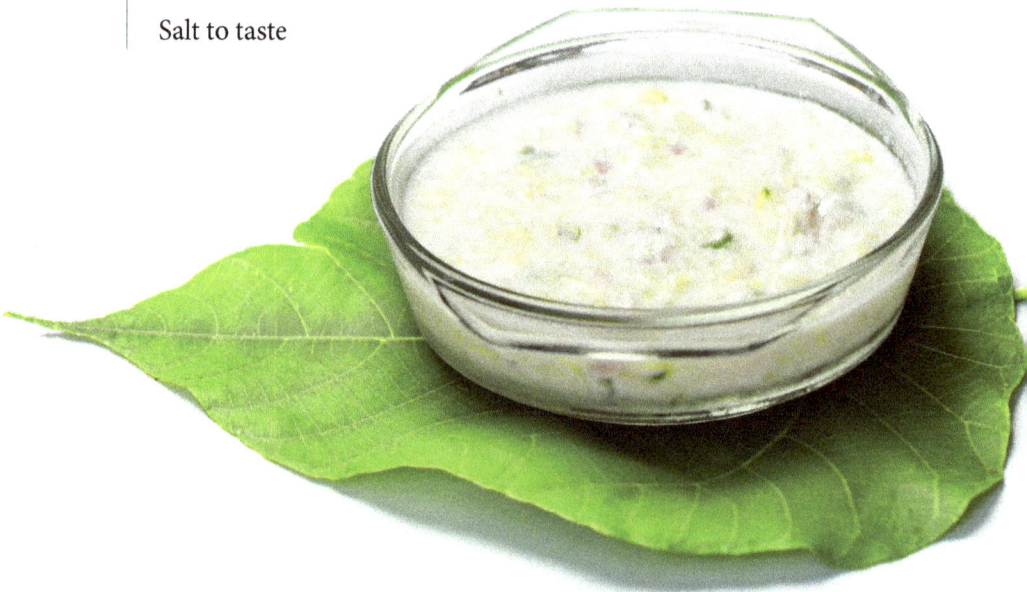

Miriam's Pacchadi (Kerala Recipe)

Ingredients

- 1 cup organic whole milk yogurt of choice
- 1 cup peeled and cubed (pea-sized) of any one or more of the following vegetables; firm cucumber, peeled and seeds removed, zucchini, daikon, turnips, beetroot, raw papaya, core of broccoli stem.
- 1 tbsp cubed (pea-sized) onion
- 1/2 tsp crushed ginger
- 1 clove of garlic, crushed
- 1 dried, red chili pepper, broken in half leave whole if sensitive to spicy foods)
- 1/2 tsp mustard seeds
- 1/4 tsp of fenugreek seeds, lightly crushed
- 1/4 tsp cumin, very lightly crushed
- 1/2 tsp turmeric
- 5-10 curry leaves if available (replace with 1 tbsp chopped cilantro if curry leaves not available)
- 1 tbsp coconut oil, or oil of choice
- Salt to taste

Process

- In a separate dish, add yogurt, salt, turmeric and mix with a whisk. Add small amount of cold water to get the mixture to a milky liquid consistency.
- In a separate dish, cook vegetables, onions, garlic and ginger and half of curry leaves (at this stage do not use cilantro if you are using cilantro instead of curry leaves) in 1-3 tbsp of water for 2-4 min until mixture boils. Add salt to taste. Cover and turn off heat. Keep aside.
- Heat oil in a medium saucepan or wok and lower heat and add mustard seed, fenugreek, red chili and cumin and remaining curry leaves to oil and lower heat to medium, until mustard pops.
- Lower heat to minimum and place the cooked vegetable mixture into the oil and mix thoroughly.
- On very low heat, add the diluted yogurt (in the first step above), and stir continuously for 1-4 min making sure the mixture is only lukewarm so that the diluted yogurt does not curdle. Turn off heat. Keep open until cooled.

Serve over hot rice, with other vegetable, fish or meat.

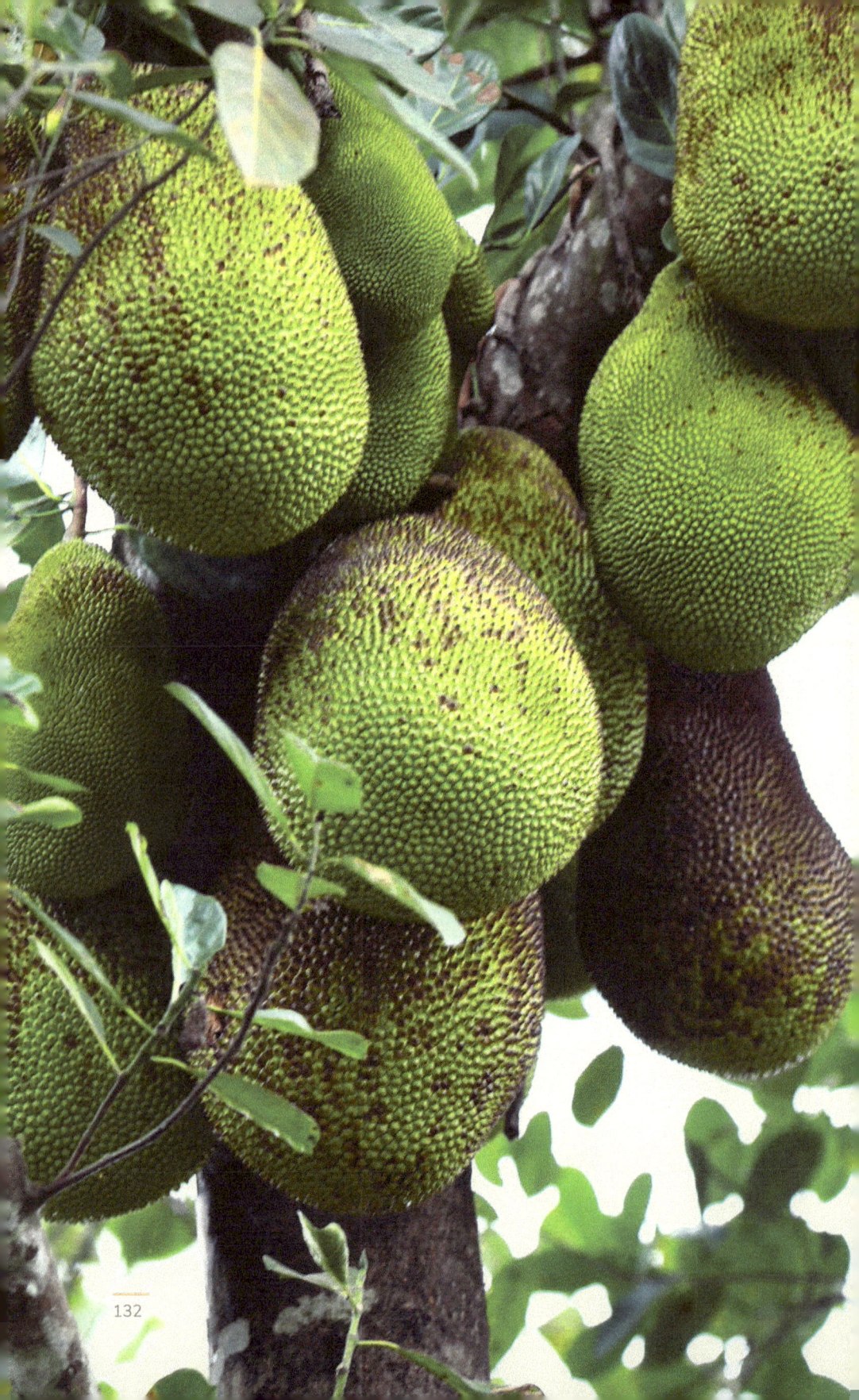

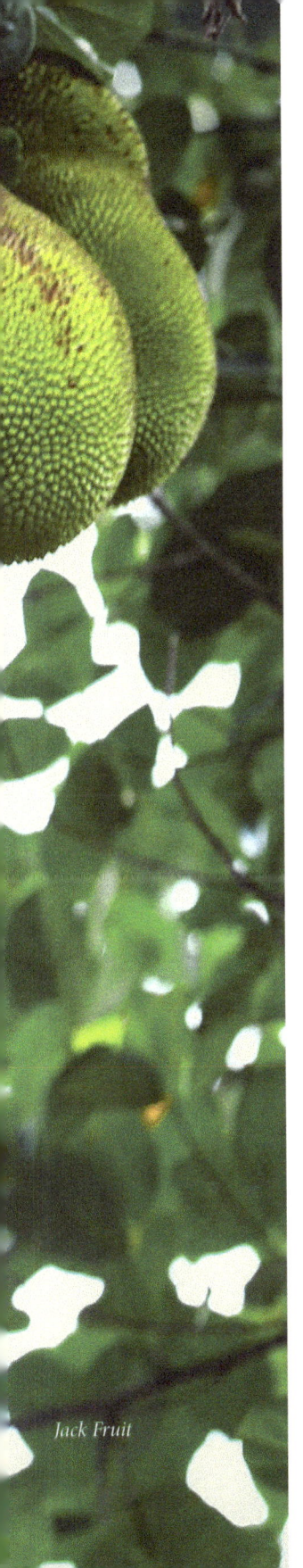

Jack Fruit

SNACKS

JACKFRUIT FLAVORED RICE CAKES
Chakka Kumbel

The first time you spot a jackfruit, or *Chakka,* hanging from a tree trunk, you are amazed. Jackfruits can weigh from 5 kg to 50 kg or more. Sporting a spiny, leathery skin, these large and lumbering, round-edged, edible growths erupt directly out of the trunk of the tree. As the tree ages and as the branches are able to support the weight of the fruit, many more of these delicious giants appear in the canopy, making them a challenge to harvest.

Jackfruits tend to appear close to the ground, almost at root level. The way they hang precariously on short stems, holding each bulky fruit firmly, reminds one of prehistoric landscapes. The tree's oval, shiny leaves are surprisingly diminutive relative to the disproportionately large fruit. The tree itself can grow quite tall, sprouting lush, glossy foliage, extending itself into a flowing canopy that can easily comfort the weary with the coolest of shade on a hot summer day. The broad, thick trunks are able to provide excellent lumber for building houses and making furniture, so much so that families became accustomed to holding on to a tree like a bank deposit, sacrificing it only in time of dire financial need, or to construct a new dwelling. Meanwhile, the tree's produce served as a centerpiece for the lush, tropical fruits of Kerala, and in 2018, it was officially declared the state fruit.

The trees begin to bear fruit as early as November and December, maturing in the hot months of April and May, and continuing through August. A truly unique quality of this enormous fruit is that its leathery outer covering holds a myriad of "mini-fruits." Once the almost inch-thick skin has been cut open, one finds hundreds of smooth, fleshy, yellow, sweet-smelling, mature florets, firmly tethered to their tough outer housing and surrounded by a tapestry of flat, fibrous strands. Each hefty floret holds a large seed, and every part of the fruit except its spiny exterior is edible. The inner, rugged skin, the fiber strands, the seeds, and the unripe jackfruit itself can be made into tempting curries. Most of these parts are rich in fiber, carbohydrates, small amounts of protein, and certain D and B vitamins. The sweet yellow flesh of the florets can be eaten raw (its most common use), fried as chips, or added to other sweets or wrap recipes, of which **Kumbel** is one. I inquire about the availability of jackfruit during my trips to Kerala to this day. I make sure that, if one is available, it finds its way into my kitchen.

During bygone, carefree, childhood years eating jackfruit was a delightful ritual that we youngsters awaited every time we saw a heavy fruit being carried into the back room of the house. There it would remain in a dark corner, covered with a gunny sack, until it was ripe. We eagerly checked the ripeness on a daily basis, pressing our fingers into it to see if the requisite sponginess had come about. The least hint of this type of "give," coupled with a sweet aroma in the room, would send us scurrying to alert Grandma that the time had arrived! Grandma, however, was the final authority, and unless she gave the green light, no one would dare serve this tropical gem before its time.

When, according to the matriarch's unquestionable authority, the time had arrived, we were told that we would be served our treat after lunch. We smeared our hands with coconut oil because the sap of the fruit is sticky and clings to fingers and palms, making the extraction of the delicious pulp covering each seed difficult. Applying oil made the process easy and provided the additional benefit of keeping our hands clean and smooth.

Using a sturdy, cast-iron knife, Grandma divided the fruit into triangular pieces. The inner, spongy core was cut out, allowing the florets to be separated by spreading the skin apart. The children would sit expectantly on the floor floor, waiting patiently with oiled fingers to be served. Each floret was pried off its base, and the oval, pearly seeds were squeezed out into a dish. Next, the sweet, firm flesh went straight into a number of eager mouths. After only one or two bites, the sweet, slippery flesh slid into our stomachs, leaving us yearning for an encore.

When it came to jackfruit, overeating was permitted. We were warned that, should any of us get a tummy ache, it was our own fault. The generous quantities each fruit provided, in addition to the fruit's robust fiber content, served as a laxative and cure for any abdominal discomfort, reassuring us that even an excessive intake was excusable.

Grandma had her own ancient solution to the potential problem of overeating. She taught us that chasing the fruit with a pinch of salt solved the problem. Not surprisingly, and toward the end of our jackfruit feast, one of the aunts magically appeared with spoonful of salt from which each of us sampled to rescue us from an unwelcome result.

Women were warned that a backache would result from overeating. One possible explanation that I deduced from my medical knowledge in later years was that the pressure would come to bear on the spine, caused by post-digestive overfilling of the colon after eating large quantities of the fiber-rich fruit. Nonetheless, there were more than a few women who consciously chose not to heed such warnings, preferring instead to indulge and deal with the consequences later.

When the fruit was plentiful, new dishes appeared on the menu, including mashed, young raw jackfruit, a meat-like curry from the seeds and inner skin, candy-like, fried crisp snacks, sweet meats or **halwa**, and **Kumbel,** steamed rice or cream of wheat cakes, flavored with jackfruit, jaggery, cardamom, and sometimes cumin. The dough was wrapped in a triangular shape, using leaves from a tree of the cinnamon family, known locally as the **Kumbel Tree.** When the pockets are steamed, the fragrance of the leaf infuses the house with a sweet balmy aroma, one that is permanently etched in memory.

Served mainly for breakfast or as a snack that is good any time of day, **Kumbel** was a staple in most Kerala kitchens during jackfruit season.

> *Jackfruit does not seem to be as abundant or popular as it used to be. One must make arrangements and seek it out well in advance. Majority of the fruit currently harvested is exported to the rest of India and even abroad or bought by factories to be processed and packaged. Many households cut down the trees for home and furniture building or to sell as timber. Sadly, the "jackfruit season" for households is over. Today, most people eat it occasionally as a sweet fruit or as a fried snack, packed in plastic bags and available on the go.*
>
> *Preparing **Kumbel** and other curries is a curiosity. When cultivated, the jackfruit is exported to foreign countries. The new world has discovered*

all the tropical fruits previously restricted to faraway lands. Children in Kerala have moved away from natural tastes and prefer a baked pastry, or sweets like cupcakes, rather than the remarkable and wholesome jackfruit. It is ironic that bakeries that sell almost all sugary and carbohydrate-laden snacks have popped up every few yards throughout Kerala. Once in a while, if a family wants jackfruit, they would rather drive to the mega store nearby to purchase it, prepped and prepackaged in plastic bags.

The ritual and camaraderie of eating together, especially when it comes to complicated fruits like jackfruit, which was a seasonal ritual in families during my childhood, has disappeared. Hope remains, as there is now a movement in Kerala schools to return knowledge of these gastronomic gems to the young, with elements added to the curriculum about "Ancient Wisdom." This is a step in the right direction. The fact remains that a child or teenager of today would rather see a jackfruit being prepped on YouTube, i.e., virtual reality, than actually preparing it themselves and getting their hands sticky.

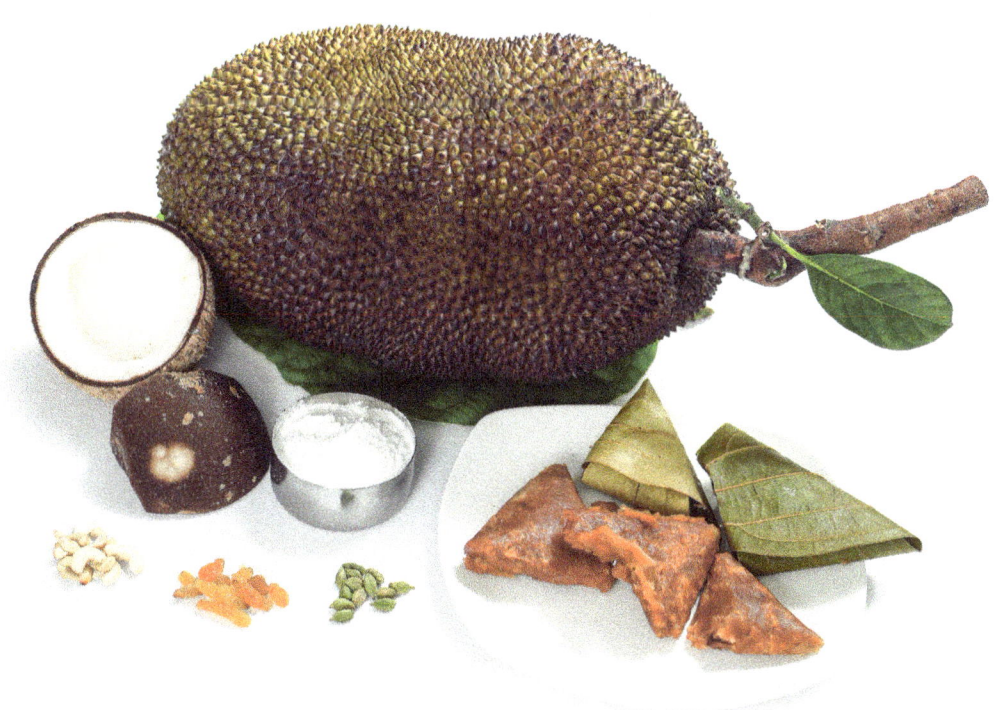

Steamed Jackfruit Wraps
Chakka Kumbel

Ingredients

2 cups cream of wheat or roasted rice flour

1 ½ cup roughly chopped sweet jackfruit pulp

3-4 cardamoms crushed roughly

½ cup of grated coconut

Salt to taste

10-15 *Kumbel* leaves (substitute with banana leaves or turmeric leaves, if available)

Process

- Mix all ingredients, slowly adding water to make a soft dough.
- Wrap the dough into a triangular form using the Kumbel leaf, and pin the stem of the leaf through the other side to keep the leaf from opening, or use a toothpick if easier.
- Steam in a bamboo or other steamer for 10-15 min.

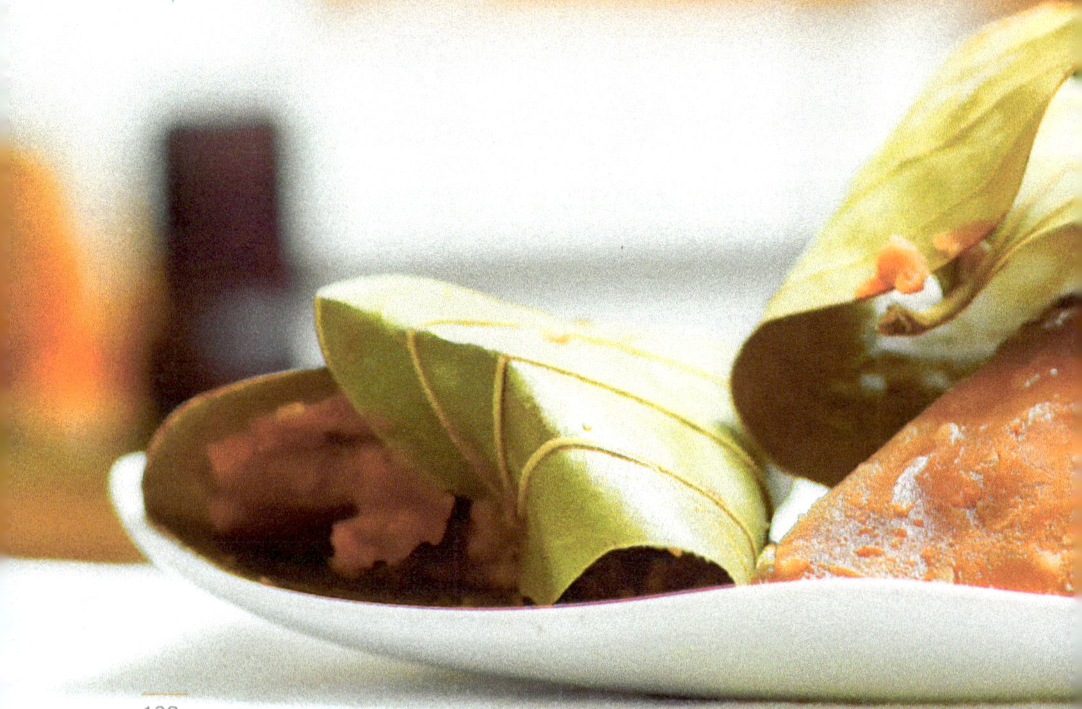

Serve hot, cold or at room temperature as a snack.

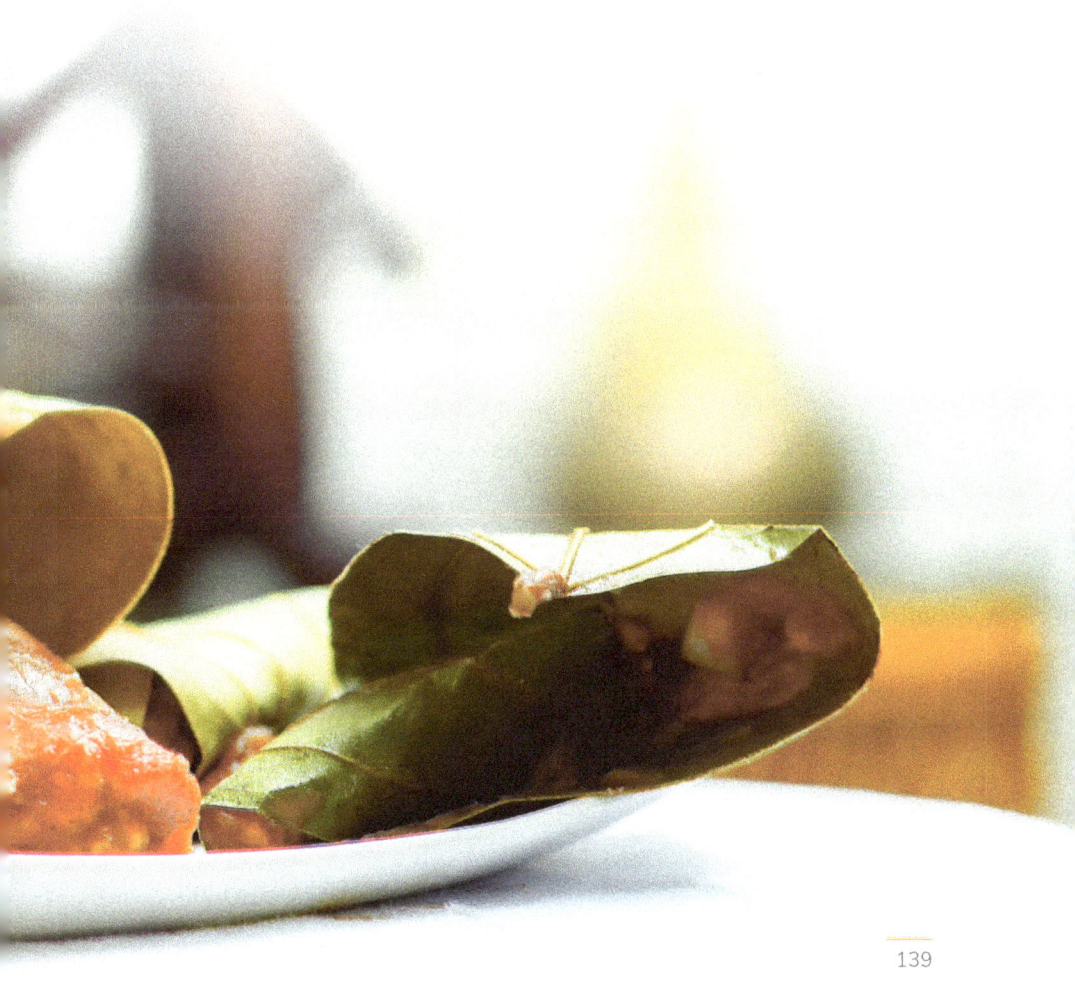

PLANTAIN FRITTERS
Etthakka Appam

I may have first encountered this magnificent morsel in my grandmother's kitchen during my childhood. On other occasions, I nibbled on one that was procured for me from the food cart of a lowly vendor that took up residence in an unassuming corner of the street. I may have even wandered across this tasty tidbit while ambling past the ramshackle eateries for the tired and weary of yesteryears. Yet another chance came when the adults would drag me along in their search for wares in the ancient "apothecary shops" of Kerala which exist to this day! These dilapidated and rickety structures have tenaciously survived for many decades, and continue to serve a loyal, local and well-established clientele. They sit somewhat out of view, deeply rooted in the soiled and unkempt rooms of ancient classic Kerala market buildings, tilting on their sinking foundations, tucked away in one of the quiet side streets untouched and unnoticed by modernity!

These curiosities, where the medicinal **Kadali** bananas hanging from the ceiling is their trademark, continue to be both a dispensary and a general store. The owner to whom the knowledge of ancient herbs and other medicinal potions has been passed down for generations, dispense remedies designed to soothe many common and transient ailments. Occasionally a homemade snack, like plantain fritters show up at one end of the counter, the wife's contribution to the business.

Kerala plantain fritters with their unmistakable savory, sweet aroma tempt and lure one into a sense of comfort and escape from the tiring and unceasing demands of everyday life. Their crispy, chewy shell, found to be alternately warm or cold when munched down on, leads to a soft, sweet, inner treat, exploding into a bouquet of buttery, and nutty flavors. When subjected to its earthy and soothing flavors, even an iPhone-empowered, modern mortal finds it unable to resist, perhaps leading to memories of their own grandma's kitchen!

Nothing, of course, could match the satisfaction I experienced when this same, treat was prepared at home, using plantains hand-picked by Grandma herself and spiked with her special touches, such as a pinch of cumin, and some spritely sesame or piquant *ajwain* seeds, added to the batter and served piping hot from the frying pan!

It has been twenty years since my most memorable encounter with **Ettakka Appam**.

Mohanan, a day laborer in his mid-thirties, along with his wife and two children, aged eight and six at that time, lived in a one-room, makeshift home, a mere twelve feet across the street. The home lay in the shadow of the towering wrought iron gates of my Kerala home, its weighty mass peering down upon their humble dwelling. I had a close relationship with Mohanan. He was one of the young laborers who, ten years earlier, worked on the construction of my home. Out of all the men involved in that job, he seemed to be the most reliable go-to person when it came to clarify any confusion about the underground plumbing lines, filtration system, or septic tanks that were tethered to the house. The location and paths of these domestic necessities, buried as they were in various parts of the property surrounding the house, were often erased from memory by pavements, paths and other structures which came after them. Mohanan was personally involved in the original excavations, and no one knew their anatomy better than him. He committed every detail to memory and has been able to retrieve that information when needed, to this day!

In the meantime, his wife Jagadamma, who occasionally worked for us as a cook, had also started a café in the miniscule space created by enclosing the verandah of their tiny home. It was there that tea and snacks could be served to laborers working nearby, who, after acquiring their lowly refreshments, would sit on the ledge of the verandah or under a nearby tree to consume them. The only furniture that would give the place the semblance of an *ad hoc* food establishment was an ancient, four-foot-high, wooden cabinet with oil smudged glass casements as windows. These looked out onto the street and displayed in them Jagadamma's simple and mouthwatering creations.

Her "display case" was equipped with four shelves, each one lined with old newspaper, displayed unevenly piled plantain fritters in the top two shelves. The remaining shelves held a smattering of several other treats, such as batter-fried, sweet lentil balls (**suhian**), deep-fried lentil cakes (**parippu vada**), and a handful of other goodies made only during holidays, in small quantities due to the cost of their ingredients. This last group typically flew off the shelves within moments of making their appearance!

When, after an outing, my car or **tuk-tuk** (three wheeled, motorized taxi) would turn into the gate of my home, I would often be met with the irresistible scent of a snack from my neighbor's cafe. On one occasion, this whiff was powerful and tempting enough to cause me to demand that my driver stop. Determined to sample Jagadamma's **Ettakka Appam**, I ignored the driver's threats and entreaties, lecturing me on the desired goods' health risks, and I gingerly stepped into the hollow of the eatery and voiced my request. Jagadamma, surprised and little taken aback, was visibly embarrassed. With a gentle shaking of her head and as noticeably disarming smile appearing in the corners of her mouth, she diplomatically refused, stating that she would rather come over to my house another day and personally cook the fritters for me. Clearly, she was concerned that the hygiene of her work space might cause me some unwanted illness.

The next morning, when the sun was barely a glimmer above the horizon, its sparkling, straight rays just beginning to spray rainbow hues over different parts of the living room wall as I sat peacefully enjoying my morning cup of **Chai** or *Chaya* as it is called in Kerala, I was surprised by a timid knock on the living room door. I opened the door curious as to who could visit at this early hour, only to be greeted by two meticulously dressed children. "Good morning!" they recited simultaneously, greeting me as they would their teachers at school and as if they had rehearsed this moment. It may even have been that their mother made them practice.

The first was a girl in a bright blue dress, donning a glittering white plastic pearl bead necklace and bangles, and the second was a slightly older boy wearing a faded but immaculately clean and ironed pair of white pants and a starched brown shirt. Their hair was still wet from their recent baths, and their eager faces were smeared with jasmine-scented talcum powder.

They gazed up at me, beaming. The little girl was holding a brown paper package, wrapped in string, through which I could see patches of oily stains, as the sweet aroma of fried plantains filled the air. I soon recognized the children as Mani and Somya, Jagadamma and Mohanan's offspring. Somya extended the package to me, her bright, shiny bracelets dangling on her wrists, and whispered to me that her Amma (mother) had made fresh plantain fritters for me, that they were still hot, and that I would not have to worry about falling sick.

Overcome with emotion, eyes brimming, I was duly humbled by this family's magnanimity. They clearly struggled for every penny they earned, yet they had opened their hearts to me, showering upon me this random act of kindness that made me feel like they cared for me. I felt joyful and content and genuinely happy. I felt that our shared existence truly mattered!

I invited the children into my living room and offered them a seat on the wicker sofa beside me. They hesitated, feeling awkward and uncomfortable in my relatively luxurious living room. Soon enough, though, they relaxed, and as more fresh tea and Britannia biscuits appeared, we ended up sharing an uncustomary morning snack of banana fritters and refreshments. Mani sank languidly into his chair but reminded himself to sit up straight whenever he got too comfortable, and Somya excitedly shared her news with me about the shimmering necklace and bracelet that her father had bought for her at the Hindu Temple Festival the previous week. At that moment, I felt that all was truly good and right in the world!

Fortunately, these handmade snacks are also often found in their original, unchanged and unadulterated form in today's high tech, gleaming, heated counter cabinets in Western-style bakeries. These bakeries strategically placed at the entrance of cavernous, new Western-style "Supermarkets" pay homage to India's unexpected sprint toward the contemporary in the last two decades.

More recently, as a testimony to this sprint to join the first world nations, the new and sparkling Kochi Airport has become known as the first one in the world to be completely powered by solar energy. It sports many modern, mall-like edifices, showcasing shining amenities, including clothing, handicrafts, essential oils, and traditional "Ayurvedic" cosmetics and remedies.

Mini-cafes have sprung up as well at airports and near newly-minted, towering glass office buildings offering Western and local fare, including plantain fritters, piled neatly one on top of another, providing one last chance for the sleep-deprived, glassy-eyed traveler to reminisce and delight in the taste of home before he sets off to the far corners of the world, seeking elusive freedoms and fortunes.

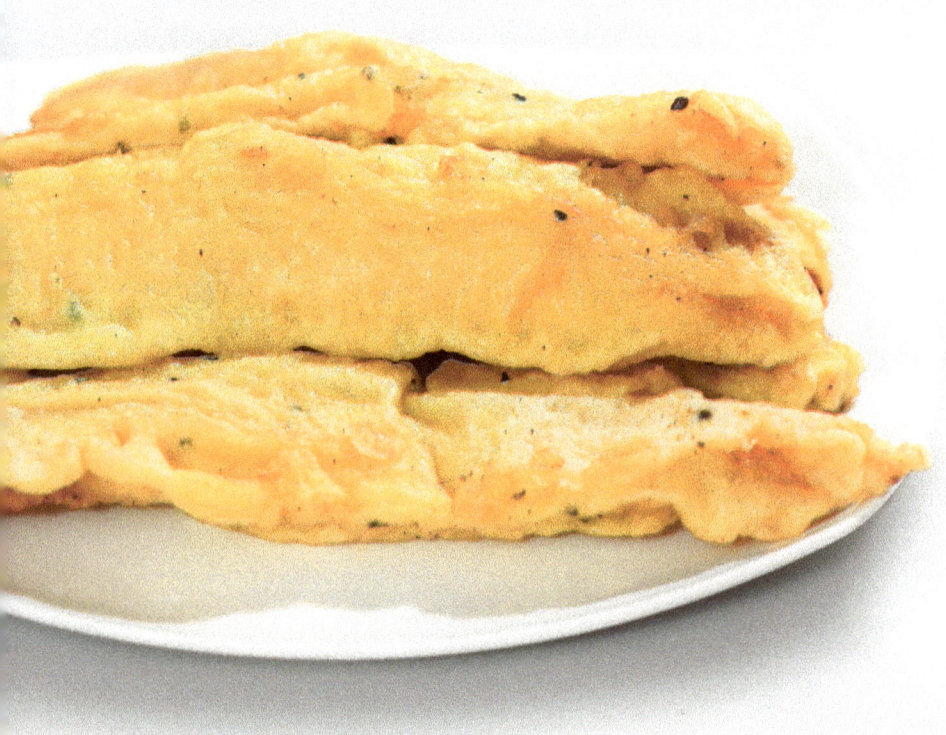

Plantain Fritters
Etthakka Appam

Ingredients

Well ripened plantains (2-3)

Organic all-purpose flour

2 tbsp rice flour

1 tsp cumin

¼ tsp turmeric

¼ tsp baking soda

1 tbsp raw sugar (optional)

Salt to taste

Enough water to create a lump-free dough

Cooking oil of choice, 1-2 cups for deep frying

Process

- Peel and cut off ends of plantain: slice crosswise into two pieces, then slice each piece lengthwise into 5 mm thick slices.
- In a separate bowl, mix remaining ingredients except oil, whisk thoroughly to avoid lumps, add water slowly until desired consistency is obtained (like pancake batter).
- Heat oil in a small or medium deep wok or frying pan.
- Dip plantain pieces into batter until completely covered. Alternatively, place all plantain pieces into batter and mix gently with hand, or two wooden spoons, so that the pieces do not break.
- Test the oil for heat by dropping a bit of batter into the oil. If it frizzles and bubbles up immediately, the oil is ready.
- Place several pieces of plantain into the hot oil at once and separate them with a spatula so that they do not stick and have enough room to cook not touching other pieces. Or place one piece at a time in oil.
- Turn once until both sides are golden brown.
- Remove with tongs, one by one, onto a plate covered with paper towel to soak up excess oil. Do not stack on top of each other while hot as they will become soggy.

*Serve hot or room temperature with tea, **chai**, coffee or as a snack by itself.*

GRANDMA'S OVERRIPE BANANA FRITTERS
Pazham Pozhi

Grandpa's land was peppered with banana palms throughout the length and breadth of its ten acres. He planted them wherever he thought the conditions were right, often along his beloved streams, near the pond, or close to where the dishes were washed outdoors. Grandpa instinctively knew where these thirsty, water-loving plants would thrive, and his wisdom paid off in large, healthy specimens that gave luscious, juicy fruit.

Grandpa also cultivated one or two larger patches of sturdy, popular banana varieties, such as plantains, and mini-varieties as well, all of which fetched good prices at the city market. These small harvests generated some much needed cash income, which was always difficult to come by in those days. The land provided most of the things that were needed to feed the family. However, cash was required to buy staples and other goods that Grandpa could not produce, and the bulk of that cash came only once a year, following an uncertain rice harvest at the close of summer.

I remember many a summer vacation at the ancestral home, when we children would spend our time locating the nectar from the unopened banana flowers that hung at the end of the sturdy stalk that held the florets, as well as ensuring that the bananas grew in neat arched rows. Picking the nectar-laden flower in the early cool and dewy morning, sucking its ambrosia-like liquid with lips pursed and expectant, and marveling as its silkiness subsequently glided along the tongue, is one of my fondest childhood memories. Looking back, I think that, as children, we set off on our nectar hunt early in the morning, because we sensed that we would only have the leftovers from the birds and the bees if we waited too long.

Kerala, with its unique ecosystem and perfect alchemy of water, humidity and soil quality, produces the most unique and diverse assortment of fruit and vegetable species seen in the world. Over a dozen varieties of bananas, each with their own unique nutritional content and flavor, have surprised and tantalized locals and visitors alike for centuries.

One miniature variety of banana, called **Pooja kadali**, is reserved specifically for Hindu Temple rituals, and is typically sold only in local, old-style, apothecary and Hindu Temple supply shops. Diminutive and unassuming, these tiny treasures have a high fiber content and are loaded with potassium, magnesium, and folate. Lore has it that these bananas even contain minute traces of gold. These endangered banana species are now being resurrected by women's groups who are successfully cultivating them to supply famous Hindu Temples like *Guruvayur Temple* in Northern Kerala.

This **kadali** is used specifically for **poojas** (ritualized, Hindu prayer ceremonies) to **Vishnu or Krishna** *and often to* **Shiva (the creator and destroyer)**, to ward off bad luck or unwanted events during periods of negative planetary influences, times of illness, and other intervals when one's physical and spiritual safety could be threatened. At the end of the ritual, the sanctified fruit is given to the devotee to consume, resulting in the cleansing of the gastrointestinal tract the following morning. This symbolically signifies the removal of harmful toxins and negative energy of any source from the body and spirit.

> *Although these fruits are used for a ritual that, on the surface, may look superstitious, the effect can be explained scientifically due to the high fiber content combined with the fruit's unique blend of nutrients, which makes it an excellent laxative. The intent of the whole ritual is to liberate the devotee from the fear of things beyond his control and empower him to take charge of his destiny.*
>
> *This practice is the result of centuries of wisdom that engages an amalgamation of spirituality, science and psychology to potentially bring about healing. It is wholly ironic that the modern mechanistic interpretation of such rituals often glibly dismisses them as nothing more than superstition, while concepts like the "placebo effect" that confound scientific explanation is intellectually palatable to the same skeptic.*

Many browning bananas remained on the banana stalk hanging from the pantry ceiling in Grandma's kitchen, after the children and the rest of the family had had their fill, prying off the ripe ones one by one for a snack. The remaining browning, overripe bananas infused the kitchen with an intensely sweet, fruity odor. This is the time when Grandma would amaze us with an unexpected and scrumptious snack.

It was time to make overripe banana fritters, to be eaten with the evening's black coffee, a perfectly paired snack.

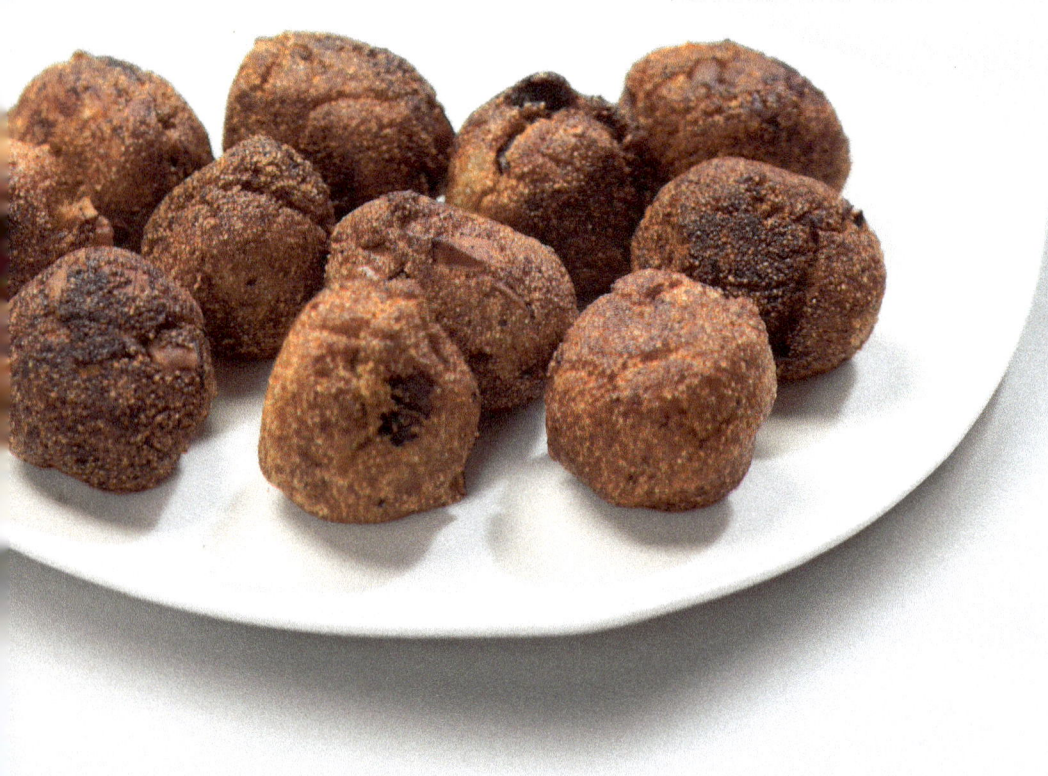

Grandma's Overripe Banana Fritters
Pazham Pozhi

Ingredients

- 2 cups cream of wheat
- 2-3 overripe bananas
- 1 tbsp sesame seeds
- 1 tbsp finely or coarsely chopped, fresh coconut (can substitute with coarsely crushed Almonds)
- ½ tsp cumin seeds
- 1 tbsp raisins
- 1 tbsp *jaggery* (brown sugar available in Indian stores) or any available brown sugar
- ¼ tsp baking soda
- Salt to taste

Process

- Crush bananas and mix all ingredients together in a large dish until thick consistency of paste is achieved (do not add water)
- Wait a minimum of two hours (can wait as much as 24 hours refrigerated)
- Heat cooking oil in a wok or deep frying pan
- When oil is hot, scoop 1/2 tbsp full of batter into oil to make small lumps to fill the surface of the oil
- Turn the fritters frequently; adjust heat to medium or low until fritters are a golden brown
- Scoop out onto paper napkin

Serve hot, warm, or room temperature with Tea or Coffee.

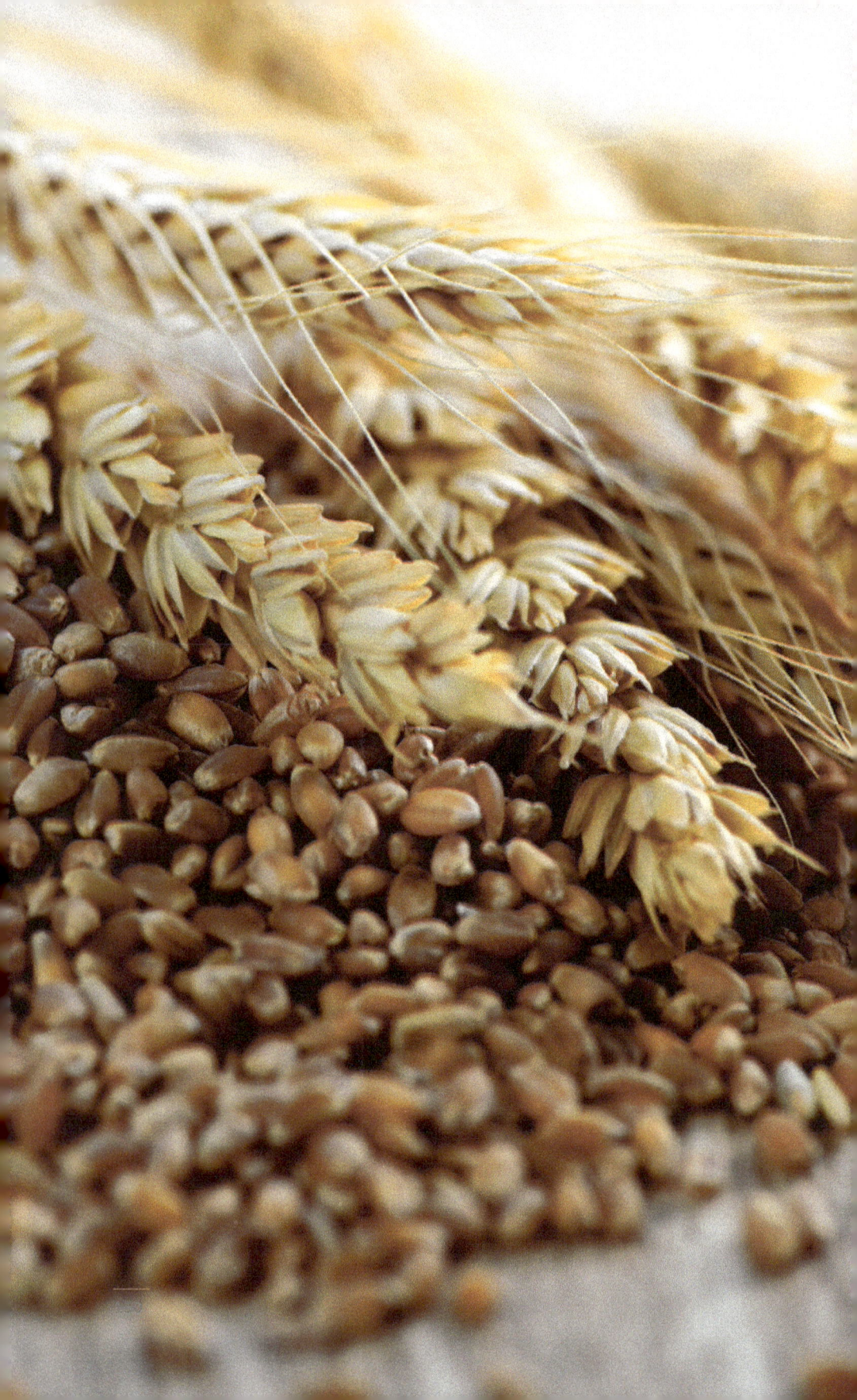

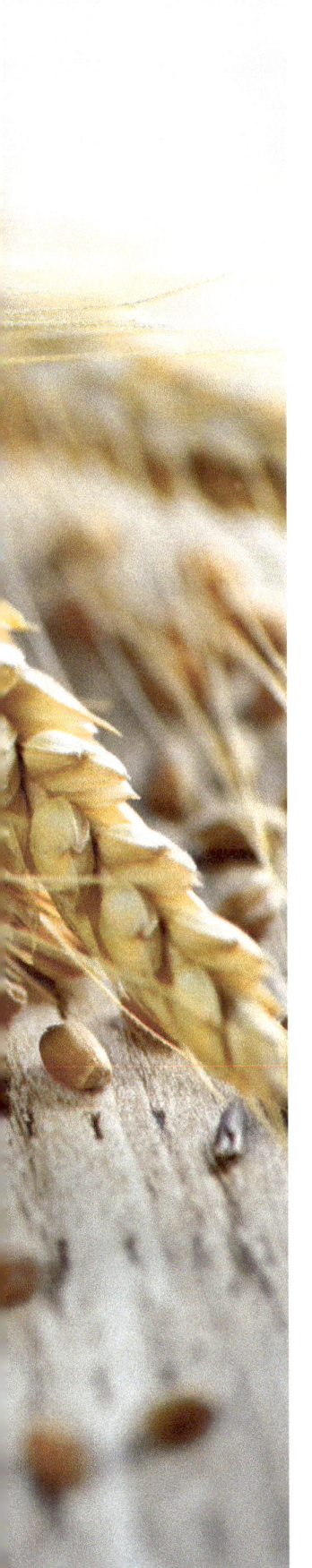

FLAT BREADS

WHOLE WHEAT FLAT BREADS
Pazham Pozhi Chapati & Triangular Parota

Whole wheat flat breads are a staple in all of India, particularly in northern India. They are essentially like whole wheat tortillas; however, the special Indian touches makes them more nutritious and creates their unique flavors.

These breads served with various assortments of Dal preparations makes them the quintessential, most affordable, nutritious and tasty meals for the rich and poor alike.

Chapati or parotta and dal was served for breakfast and dinner on most weekdays in Jabalpur when I was growing up in Northern India. Nevertheless, we children never tired of it and looked forward to this delicious fare. Served with hot Chai it made a sumptuous breakfast or served with other vegetables and pickle, it made a well-balanced satisfying dinner.

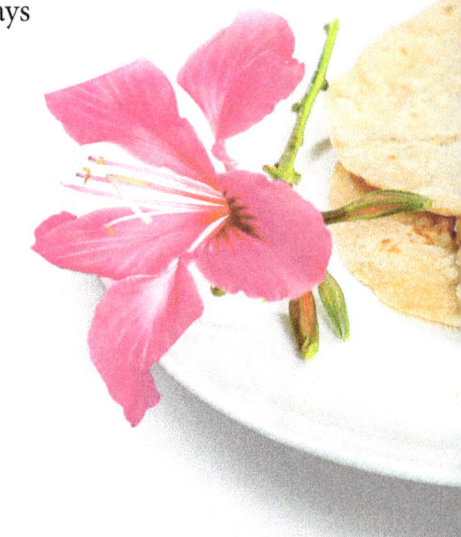

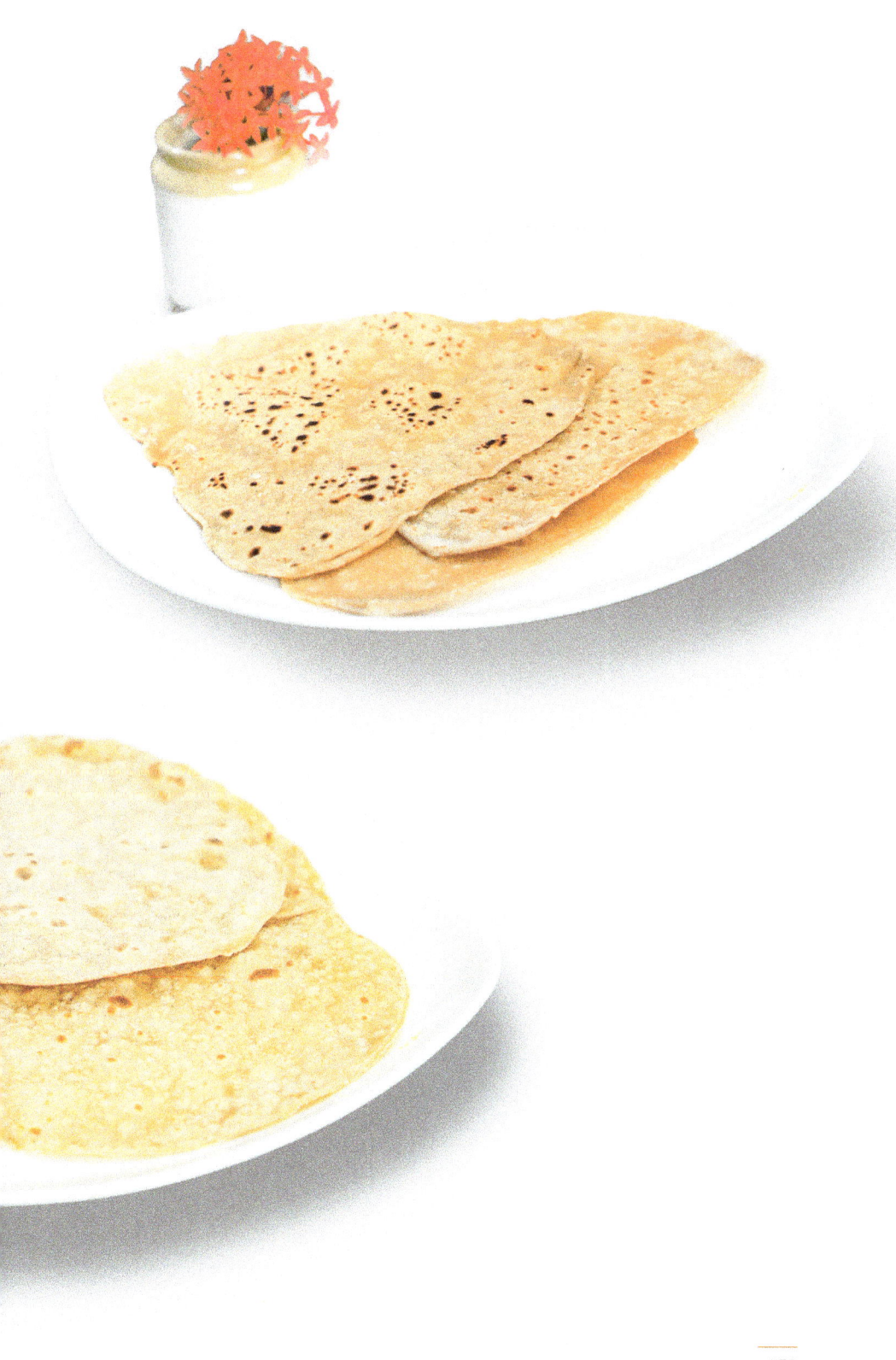

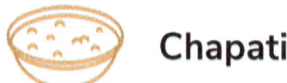# Chapati

Ingredients

> 4 cups organic whole wheat flour save ¼ cup for rolling
>
> ¼ tsp salt (adjust salt to individual taste)
>
> 2 tsp ghee
>
> ½ cup room temperature water (adjust water as needed)

Process

- In a large flat tray or mixing bowl, mix flour and salt and slowly add water, one to two teaspoons or drops at a time (toward the end) and mix and knead until dough is of a consistency to roll. Knead for 5-10 min to make soft fluffy chapatis. If a food processor is used, follow food processor instructions. Keep dough aside covered with a slightly moist cloth for 20-30 min.
- Make small lemon sized balls of dough.
- Flatten the balls with finger to palm sized patties.
- Dip the patties in dry flour and roll out evenly to 2-3 mm thickness. Lay on parchment paper on a porcelain or stainless-steel flat dish, or transfer directly to cooking griddle.
- Heat chapati tava or griddle.
- Place chapati on tava cook for 30-40 sec on one side.
- Flip chapati to other side cook for 30-50 sec and adjust the heat so that the chapati does not burn. Lightly press the surface with a wooden or metallic spatula. This makes the chapati puff out. Keep pressing the sides of the initial puffed area lightly and eventually the whole chapati will puff out. This makes the dough to be delicately roasted rendering it a special flavor. *This maneuver takes some practice and after many attempts this skill will be mastered.*
- Apply ½ tsp of ghee to one side of the chapati. While chapati is still hot and on the pan. For a lighter fare, omit the ghee

Serve with piping hot dal, vegetable and meat dishes.

 # Triangular Parota

This parotta is not the same as the classic Kerala Parota which is extremely high in calories and made with all-purpose flour or Maida, which is commonly served in Kerala and is extremely tasty but not very good for one's health.

I grew up eating the Triangular Parota, which might have been an improvised, practical version of the North Indian Ghee Parota, deemed healthier and easier to make. Universally loved, it is one of the favorite dishes of Ahimsa Retreats patrons.

Use the same dough as for chapati above

Process

- Follow the first 3 steps as above.
- Apply ¼ to ½ tsp of ghee to the rolled patty.
- Fold in two and apply a smaller amount of ghee again to the top surfaced of the folded patties. Fold again.
- Roll out the dough into a triangular shape.
- Heat chapati tava or griddle.
- Make sure heat is lowered. Cook for 40-60 sec on one side, then turn to other side and cook for 40-50 sec lightly pressing the surface with a wooden or metallic spatula. This makes the parota fluff out. Keep pressing the sides of the initial fluffed area lightly and eventually the whole parota will puff out.
- *This takes some practice and after many attempts this skill will be mastered. Do not worry if the parota does not fluff out. Parota might not fluff out as easily as the because the parota is heavier and has more layers than the chapati. It is cooked when the sides are browned and dotted with a spray of darker spots and a nutty aroma of wheat and ghee fills the kitchen.*

Serve with piping hot dal, vegetable and meat dishes.

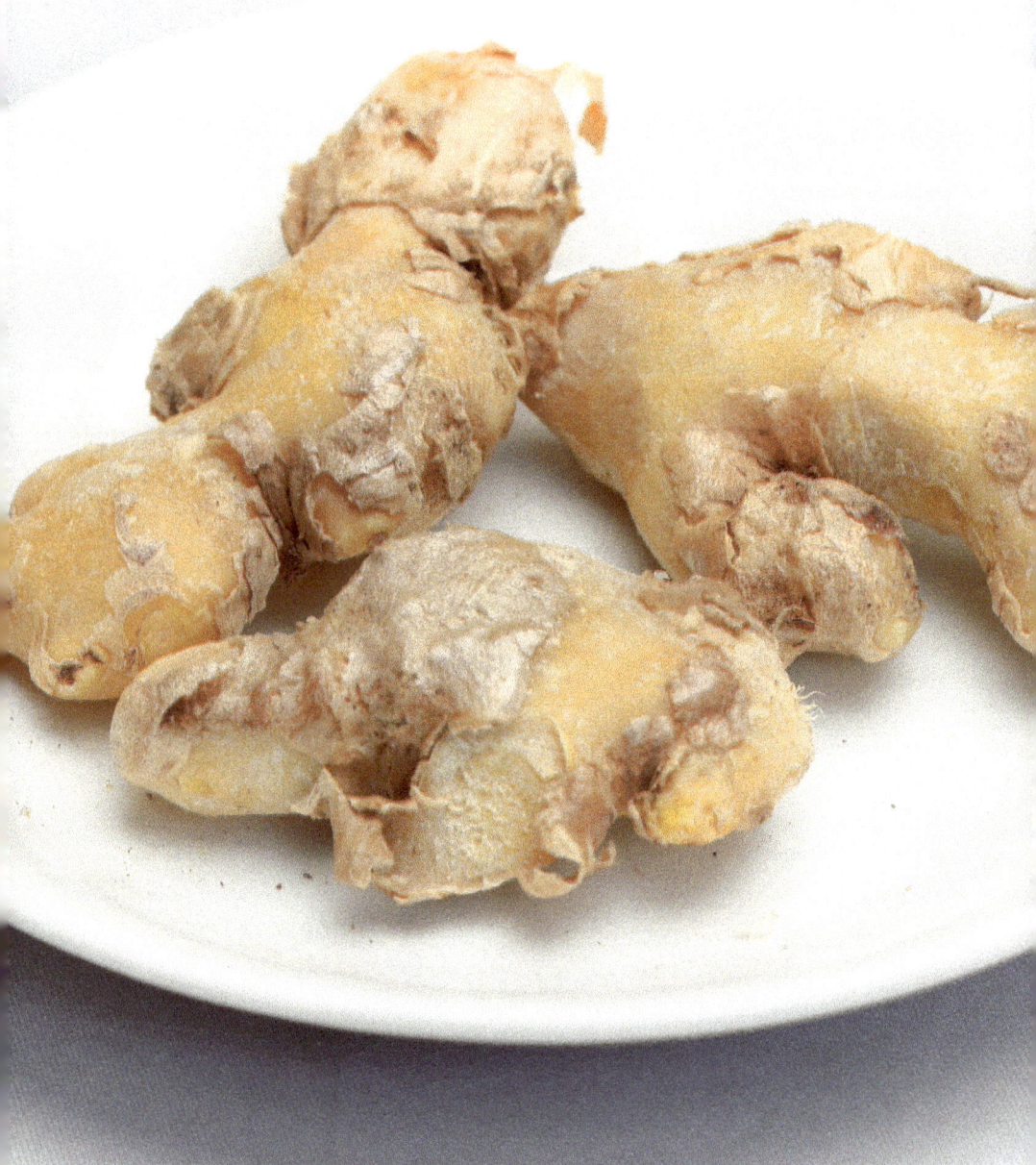

CHUTNEYS, SAMBAR & GINGER RELISH

GINGER RELISH
Ingi Curry

I have added this recipe to the book by popular demand. Of the groups that visit Ahimsa retreats Anne-Marie and her groups from the UK have been the most frequent bi-yearly visitors. Usually most of my British guests prefer their meals to be only lightly spicy. Ginger Pickle, however, piqued their curiosity, and they dared to try it once with their chapati and dal. To my surprise, after taking a tiny amount on the tip of their forks and placing it into their mouth, their faces beamed with pleasant surprise. Ignoring the spicy heat, they dared to place a teaspoon full on their plates. In no time, they were sampling more and asking for ginger pickle at lunch and dinner every day.

I started writing this book on the request of Ahimsa Retreat guests, who wanted to re-create the tastes back in their own homes. This book, of course, turned out to be more than that. During one of my transcontinental telephone calls, it was Anne-Marie who reminded me again, "You do have the Ginger Pickle recipe in there, don't you?" I had not thought of it at all. So thanks to her, here it is!

> *Ginger is one of the age-old medicinal and cooking herbs used in Ayurveda. It is most commonly used for nausea, heartburn and indigestions of any kind. A simple ½ tsp of crushed ginger with a little honey or by itself will immediately relieve and soothe all of these ailments. Repeat the dose several times and you will feel restored and ready for your next meal.*

Ginger is also anti-inflammatory and helps coughs, colds, and chest congestion. Ginger paste by itself or in combination with other herbs like turmeric can be topically applied or taken internally for musculoskeletal pain, i.e. muscle or joint pains.

Combining ½ tsp of Ginger Pickle to any meal ensures excellent digestion of the meal consumed.

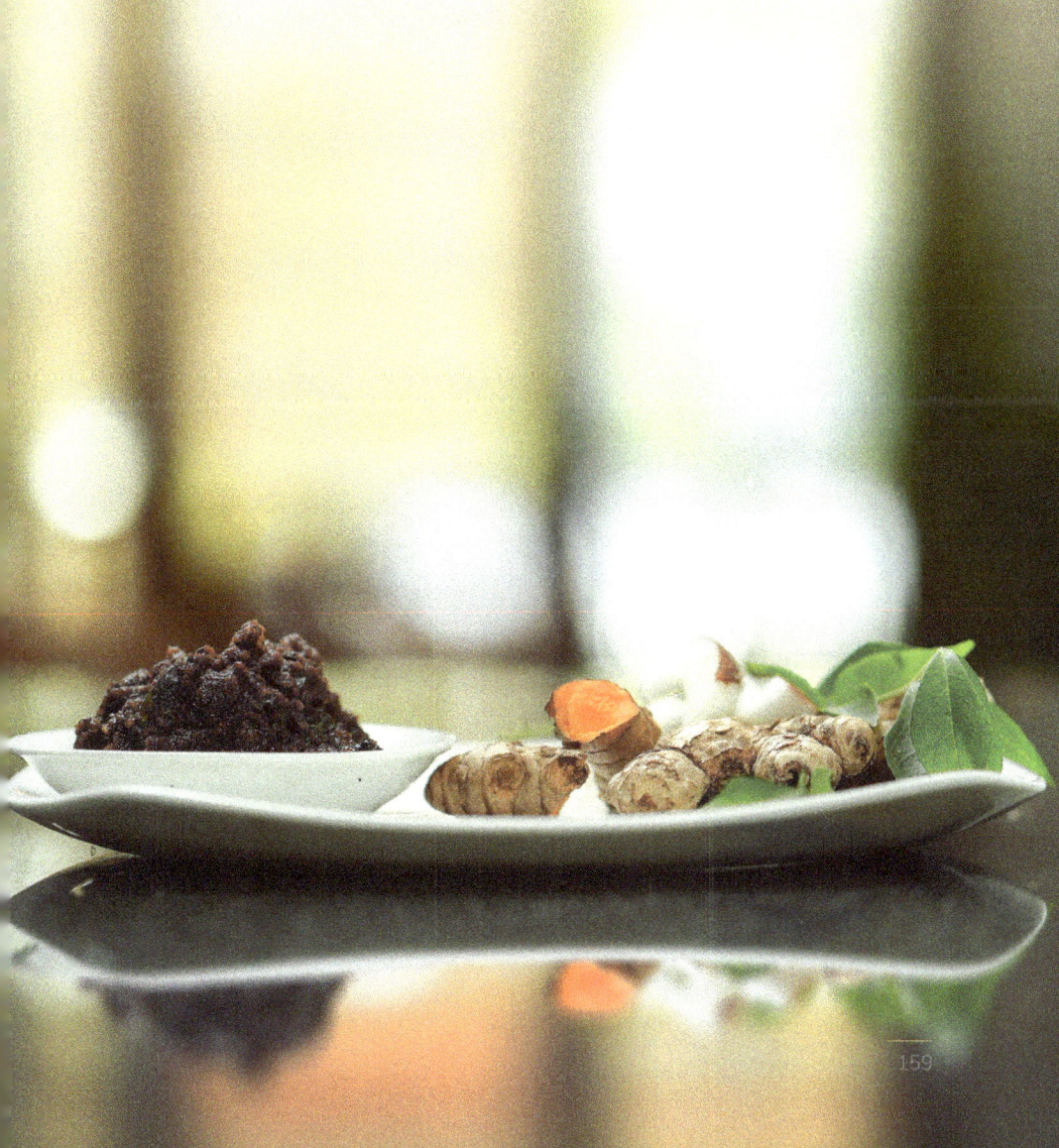

Ginger Relish

Ingredients

2 cups, peeled and finely steps diced fresh ginger root (may use food processor for this and for 2 & 3 below)

1 medium-sized green chili, deseeded and diced finely

10-15 curry leaves finely diced

2-3 tsp of coconut or sesame oil

1 tsp of mustard seed

½ tsp of hot chili powder

¼ tsp of turmeric

⅙ tsp (or 2-3 dashes) of asafetida

½ tsp of brown sugar

½ tsp of tamarind paste* (available in Indian stores)

¼ to ½ tsp of salt to taste

*Peeled, de-seeded, compressed tamarind cakes are also available in Indian stores. Pry off or cut out 1-2 tsp of this, soak in ¼ cup of hot water. One can use 2 tbsp of the tamarind water instead of the paste for a more authentic taste.

Process

- Heat oil in a small skillet or sauce pan.
- Place mustard seeds in hot oil until they pop. Keep partially covered or covered with mesh so that the seeds do not pop out over the counter.
- Lower the heat to medium and place ginger chili and curry leaves into the oil, stirring constantly for 2 min.
- Sprinkle contents of the pan with chili powder, turmeric, asafetida, and a small amount of salt. Stir constantly until well roasted.
- Pour tamarind water into the contents.
- Cook on medium heat with intermittent stirring for 8-10 min.
- Add brown sugar* and additional salt to taste.
- Remove from heat. When contents are cooled, transfer to a clean, dry glass jar with vacuum lid if available.
- *If the dish is found to be too spicy hot, more brown sugar can be added to make the dish more palatable.

Contents will last unrefrigerated for 2-4 weeks if care is taken to only use dry clean spoons to serve, or refrigerate to last longer.

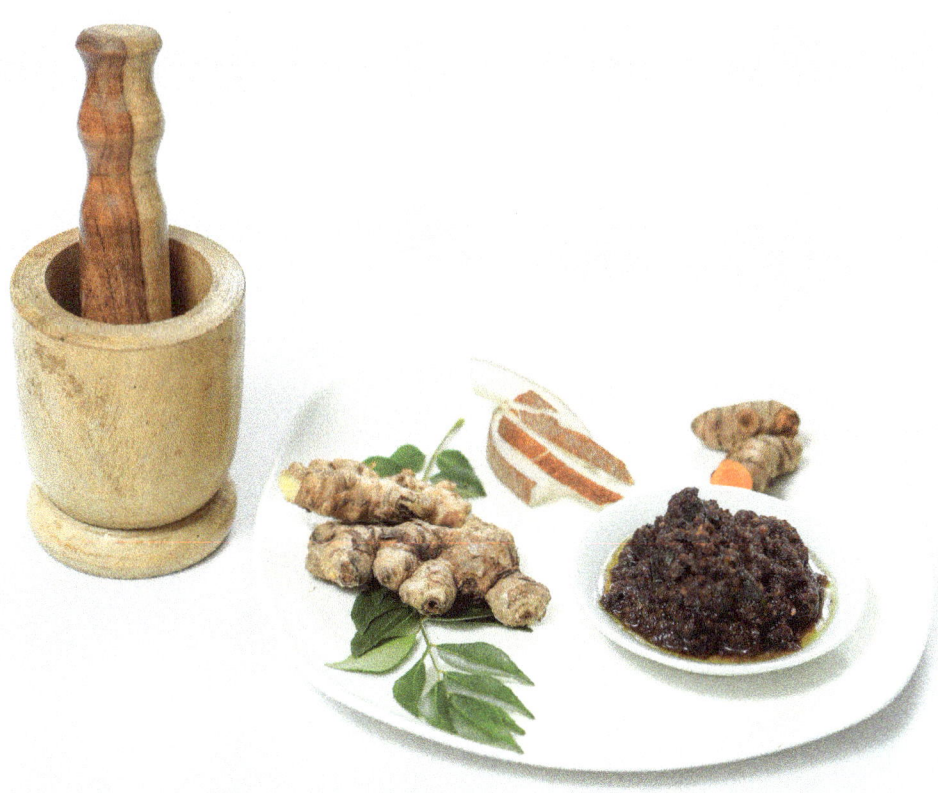

 # Coconut and Mint Chutneys

Ingredients

Grated fresh or frozen coconut 2 -3 cups

Fresh grated ginger root ½ tsp

Tamarind paste or fresh Tamarind ½ tsp

4-5 fresh curry leaves (optional)

½ medium sized red dry chili, or fresh green chili

Salt to taste

Water ¼ cup or as needed

Process

- Place all ingredients in a blender or food processor and add small amount of water to make a coarse paste.
- Add 1tbsp fresh chopped mint leaves to above ingredients and follow the same purpose to make Mint Chutney.

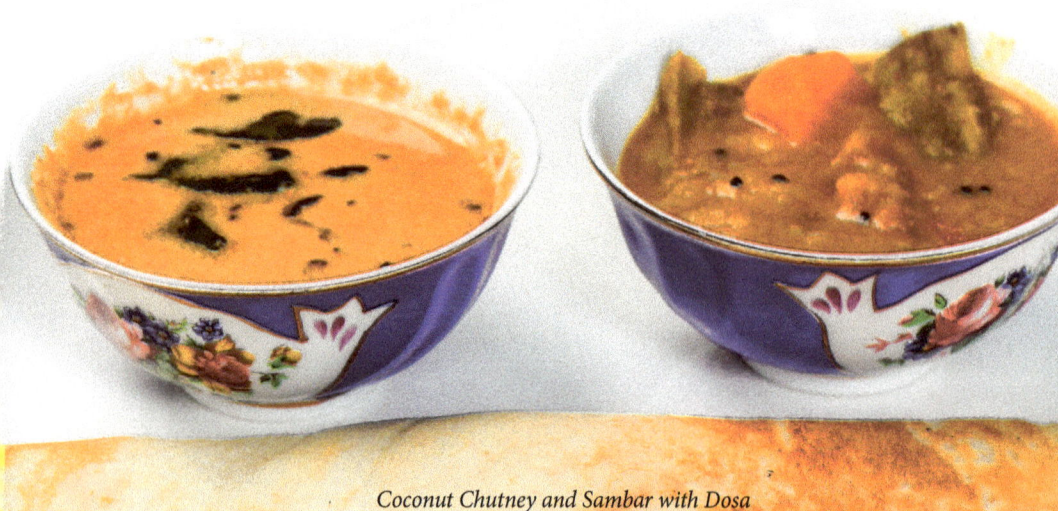

Coconut Chutney and Sambar with Dosa

Sambar

Ingredients

- ½ cup each of 2-4 varieties of your favorite vegetable of choice, (e.g. Daikon, pumpkin, string bean, potato) Cut into large cubes or slices
- ½ cup cubed tomatoes
- ½ cup Toor Dal (lentil)
- 2 tbsp of oil of choice
- ½ cup coarsely cut onions or peeled small shallots
- 2 cloves of garlic crushed or diced
- 1 tsp fresh grated ginger
- 3 whole dried red chilies
- 5-10 curry leaves
- 1 tsp mustard seed
- ½ tsp Turmeric
- 3 tsp Sambar Masala
- 1 tsp of Tamarind Paste
- Salt to taste

Process

- Boil the vegetables in (item 1 above) in ½ cup of water until most of the water is gone.
- Wash Toor Dal thoroughly and cook in deep saucepan with 1-2 cups of water for 20-30 min until cooked. Bring dal to a boil, then lower the heat and cook covered. Dal does have a tendency to spill out of the saucepan and requires opening lid and stirring every few minutes. Sometimes, more water may need to be added to bring the cooked dal to a well-cooked almost creamy consistency.
- In a separate deep saucepan heat oil.
- Add mustard seeds, red dry chilies and curry leaves until mustard starts popping. Add 2-3 dashes of Asafetida into the hot oil.
- Then lower heat to medium and add garlic and ginger and onions. Sautee on medium heat until the onions are soft.
- Add sambar powder, turmeric and stir well on low-medium heat for 3-5 min.
- Add tomatoes and stir for 2-3 minutes min.
- Add cooked vegetables to the pan and mix well.
- Add cooked Dal to the mixture adding some water if needed to bring it to the desired consistency of a mildly thick soup.
- Add Tamarind and mix well.
- Add salt to taste.
- Simmer in covered dish in low heat for 10-15 min.

Serve hot over rice and with Dosa or Idli.

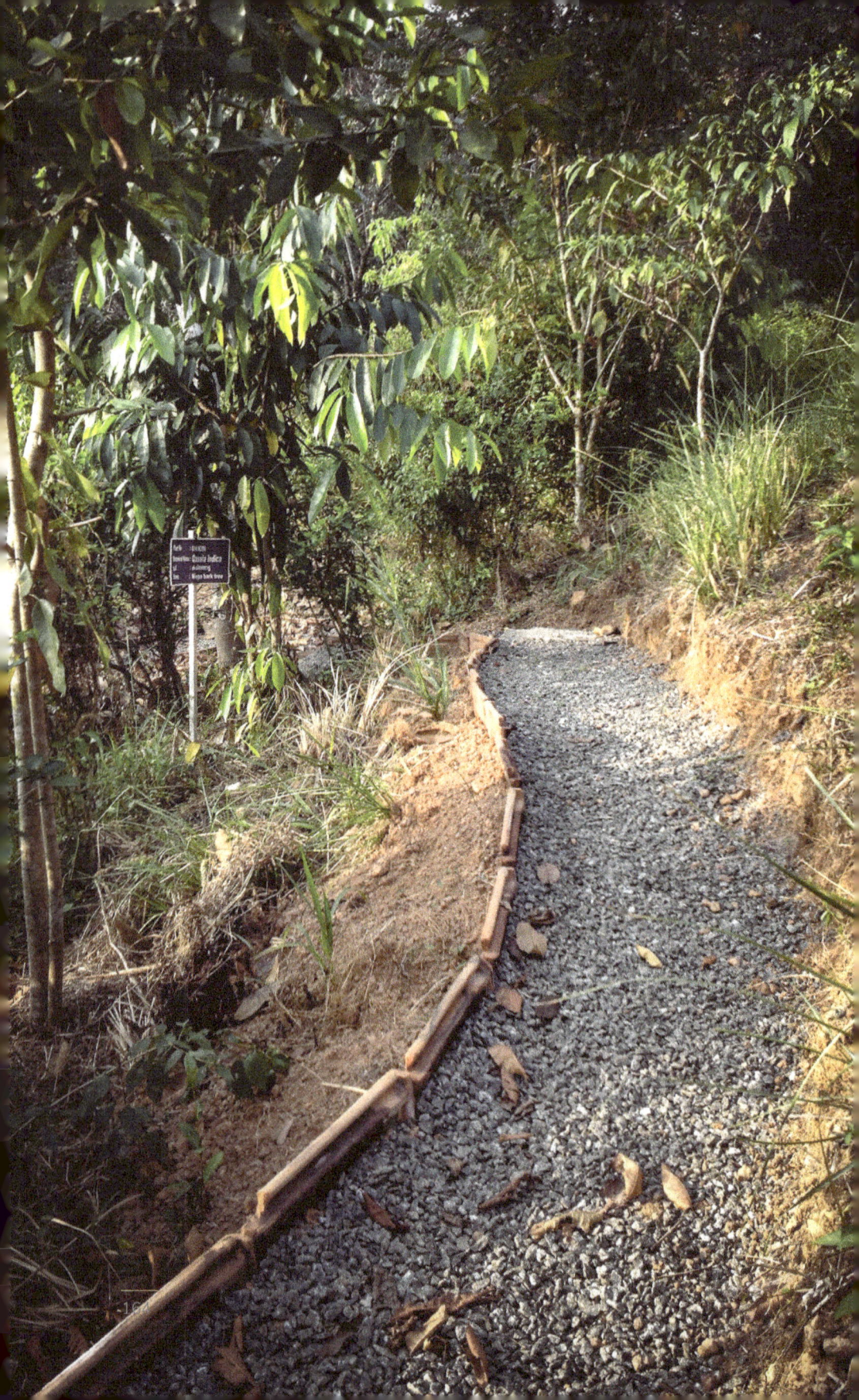

THE STORY OF AHIMSA

The community service volunteers had just left that morning in 2009—twelve students, 11th and 12th graders, two parents, a teacher and Karl. Karl was a veteran parent leader who faithfully volunteered year after year to organize and accompany the group. The group came from a small high school in Portland, Oregon, a school my son attended, thousands of miles away. They traveled to Hope Charities in Kerala, India for two weeks of community service. The students, who were selected after a stringent selection process, received a year of preparation including cultural sensitivity training, learning about India and raising funds.

With a combination of the community's desperate need and the miraculous good will of friends, I formed Hope Charities, a 501c3 charitable organization, in 2001. Funds were raised and refurbished equipment arrived from an NGO in Portland. I opened the clinic twenty years before I thought I would retire. After my retirement, I intended to volunteer every year for a few months in the one room clinic, but the universe had other plans. The Universe did, however, bring us Dr. Shashi, a soft spoken, ego-less local family practitioner who volunteered to run the clinic. This gentle soul, well known in the community for treating poor patients without charge, refused compensation for his services. He was eventually obliged to accept compensation as a condition of his employment.

The charity served about 550 families, providing them with free outpatient healthcare and educational scholarships for the children. We built a few homes, built bathrooms, and refurbished water supply and other essentials for needy families as funds allowed. In 2008, we also established the Women's Vocational Center to teach some of the women sewing and other income generating skills.

Yearly for half a dozen years, Karl and his entourage raised funds for the clinic and arrived with suitcases full of medical supplies, books and sewing supplies. They then shared a few days in service of the disadvantaged. The visitors were ready to immerse themselves in a new world. They were consistently surprised at how delightful they found the customs and traditions of a different culture. The students, while helping the community, participated in a cultural exchange program during which they visited and spent time in local schools, made new friends, and learned about the community's families. At the school, the exchange was highlighted with a cultural program which showcased folk dancing, songs, and debates involving the social and economic norms of the East and West.

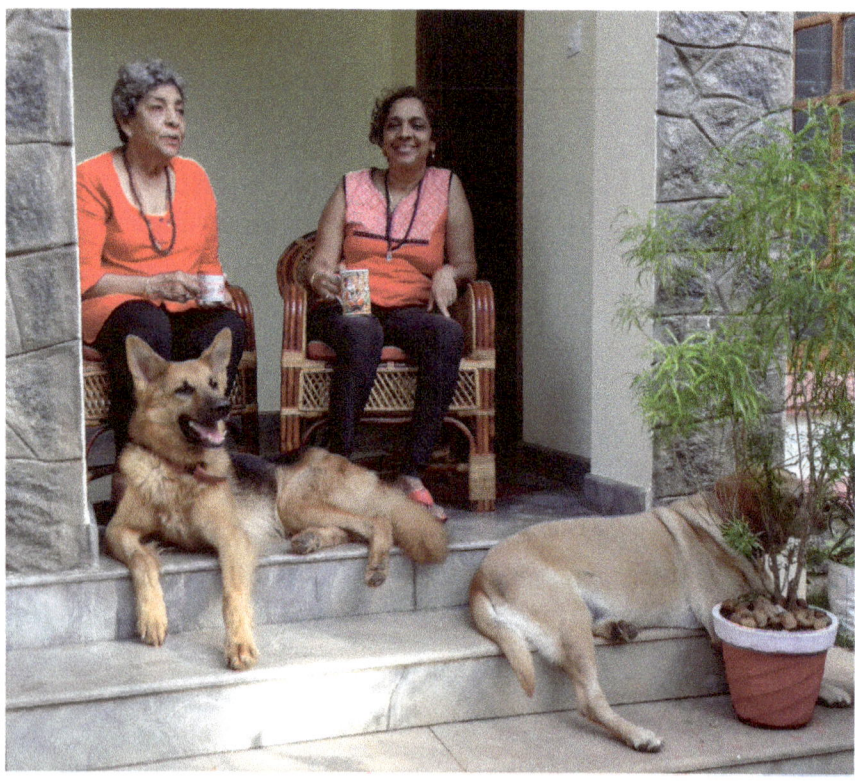

The Author, Swaran Masi, Jacky and Rosy enjoying a morning cup of tea at Ahimsa

In the Hope community, the whole experience culminated in the Hope Charities Community Service Day when all the volunteers dressed up in Indian attire for an afternoon of dancing to regional and Bollywood and Hollywood music, feasting and fun. Invariably, both sides learned that the benefits of the community service were mutual and that they were not that different from each other. In an earlier year, during a feedback session with students back in Portland, one of the students burst into tears. At the Hope Clinic, she explained, *"For the first time in my life, I could feel and as soon as I landed back in JFK, I became numb again…. I wish I could bring that feeling back"*. We adults were speechless, unable to respond, wondering where we were going wrong in the protected world of comfort we had created for our children.

One particular year, Karl and his group left the house late afternoon. The students were unusually somber, some of them tearful as they made themselves comfortable in the mini bus taking them to the airport. The previous year, we had a special parent volunteer, Susie. She was a mother in her mid-forties who accompanied her daughter as part of the group. Susie was known for her beaming smile and consistency with students. She could get them to do almost anything without losing her disarming smile. That year, 2009, the silence in the bus was particularly palpable. During this trip the students worked for a whole week putting the finishing touches on a one room addition to the original clinic building. They painted the interior walls and created colorful marine murals. A few hours before they embarked on the bus, Karl conducted a ceremony dedicating the new room to Susie. She had passed away a few months earlier. The group silently stood in front of the building as Karl affixed a little plaque in her memory over the door frame of the new addition.

A few months after Susie's death, her daughter wrote to me to thank me for the Hope experience that she and her mother had. She said that during her mother's last few weeks, when she was sent home on Hospice, the only thing that would make her smile were the videos that she had taken during their time at Hope Clinic. Later, a mutual friend mentioned that Susie requested that she be buried in the green silk sari that she wore at the Hope Charity Community Service Day.

After the bus left that day, I retreated to my room upstairs. The sun was slowly gliding towards the horizon, as the rays reflected off the tops of the rubber trees on the adjacent property. Just a few days before their departure, we had received the jarring news that the adjacent 2.5 acres of rubber plantation was bought by an Indian expat living in Chicago. He had not only procured the land, he also already had the permit to quarry the land for soil and rock, which would earn him a lot of money in short order.

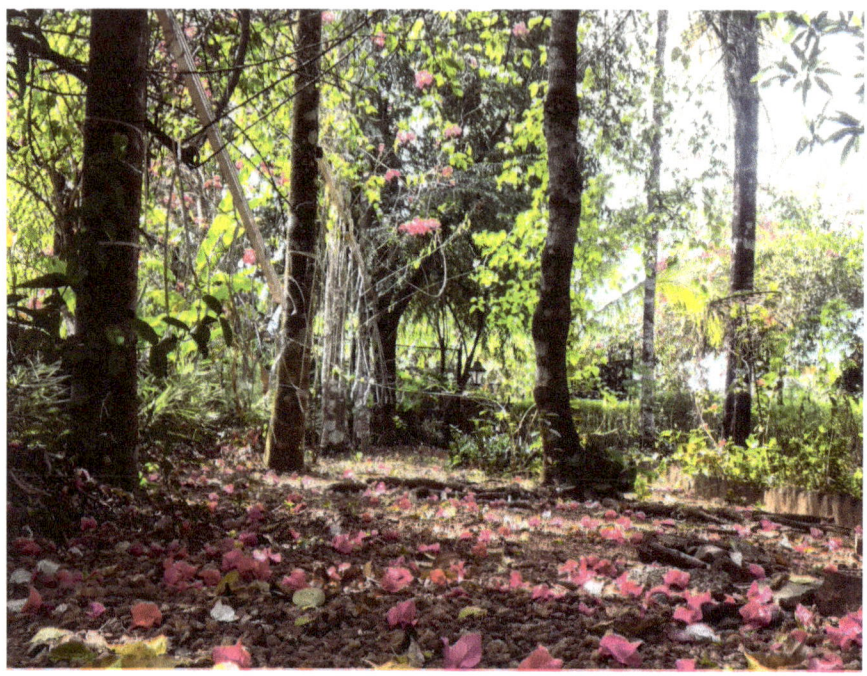

The effects of an earlier quarry on the other side of this endangered property was already causing havoc in the neighborhood. The gaping mouth of this older quarry, over 500 meters deep, had swallowed everything in its path, turning into a red muddy lake when it finally hit the deep-water aquifers that sustain the landscape. Land along the edge of the quarry fell into this demonic chasm, bringing down trees and nibbling away at the neighboring acreage. Downhill, drinking water wells upon which the locals depended on began drying prematurely during the summer, causing existential suffering for families who lived downhill. This is ongoing. The remaining land that makes up this hill consists predominantly of rubber plantations, peppered with wild cashew nut trees and punctuated by ever-shrinking plots of vegetable, tapioca and pineapple cultivation and a few scattered coconut trees.

All these properties including ours are on the slopes of a hill called **Kakkunnu.** My maternal ancestral home and the homes of a dozen close and distant relatives stand within a half mile radius. My mother and her next of kin, and my cousins and I, spent many enchanted afternoons playing on this hill top during summer holidays. From this vantage point, the surrounding vistas of lush green mountain ranges could be scanned unobstructed while we ate wild berries and cashew apples and singed our fingers while roasting cashew nuts over an open fire. All the while, our pleasure was fanned by the cooling breeze from the backwaters and lowlands that lay beyond before merging into the Arabian Ocean.

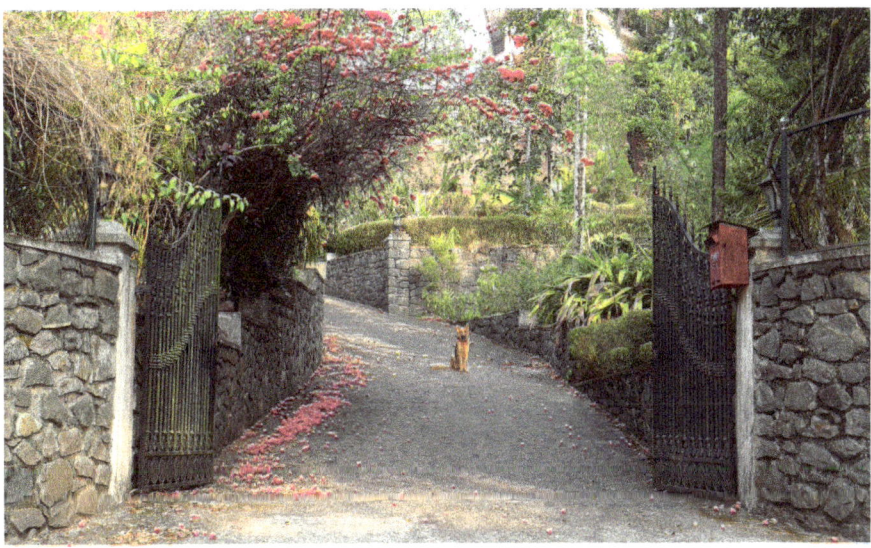

Another quarry swallowing up a significant part of this hill would mean total destruction of this pristine ecosystem. Though maligned by the monoculture of rubber cultivation, this land miraculously still holds the seeds of biodiversity. In only a few years of mindful tending, it could return it to its former magnificence.

These lands possess the ingredients to manifest the invaluable treasures of the Malabar Coast. The original inhabitants of these hills and mountains include rare, venerated trees like **rudraksha** (Hindu prayer bead tree), sandalwood, and banyan trees, sought after timber like mahogany and teak. There are also succulent tropical fruits like jackfruit, varieties of mangoes and banana, and the sweetest and most fragrant pineapple. There are also to exotic vegetables like bitter gourd, snake gourd, Chinese string beans and Moringa Pods (also called Drum Sticks) and precious nuts such as cashews, almonds, black pepper, nutmeg, coffee and cocoa. Among these faunae, the most sought after are exquisite spices including cinnamon, cloves, cardamom, ginger, turmeric and hundreds of species of medicinal plants. Spice traders from far and wide traversed the Silk Road and the Arabian Sea for thousands of years to partake of this treasured abundance.

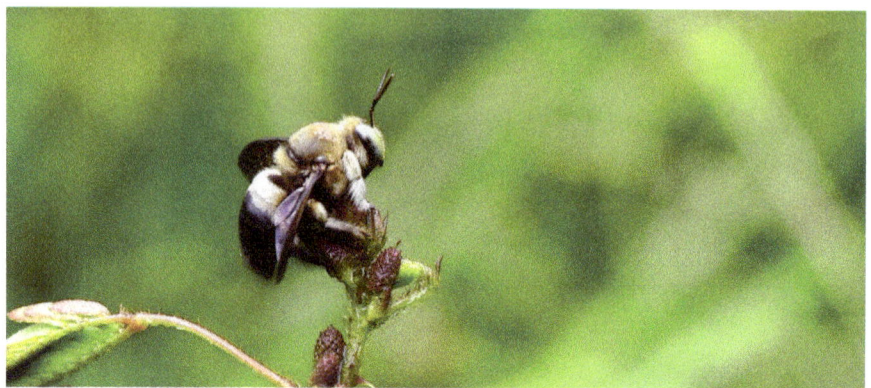

Yet, within a matter of a few decades, we have lost our way. We now wander around blindfolded, wielding swords of destruction. Businesses, consolidating to behemoths, aided by technology, have replaced utility with profitability, sacrificing sustainability to planned obsolescence and belligerent profit. As a species, we have sacrificed the meaningful pursuit of life's essential needs on the altar of wants, intoxicated with the reckless seeking of profit, appearance, and hedonism. The genuine, grounding and rigorous has been replaced with the hollow, transient and convenient. Humanity and human interactions have metamorphosed from transformational to transactional with the value of everything being calibrated only on the scale of its monetary worth.

Consequently, no one except the wise and the elderly seemed to be concerned when the vegetable and tapioca beds are erased to make room for row after row of **Hevea brasiliensis,** rubber tree saplings. After patient waiting of a half dozen years, the rubber harvests can triple incomes without much work. Previously, hardworking landowners and family members, rich and poor, men who worked the land and women who prepared and preserved the product of the land could now afford to sit in front of a television, enjoying foods they bought, prepared and packaged in the department stores, arriving from neighboring states and faraway places. Now, even walking would mean that you would be seen as someone who could not afford a car or to hire a tuk-tuk.

The Hope Clinic staff, over the sixteen years of operations, have noticed the trend of diagnosis shifting from diseases of poverty like malnutrition and infections to diseases of affluence and sedentary lifestyle like diabetes, high blood pressure and obesity, previously rare in these communities. In the meantime, the myriad flora and fauna languish, their seeds buried, unborn, choked by the tentacles of the of the gargantuan root systems of the rubber trees which blanket large tracts of land throughout Kerala. The treasured plants, birds, butterflies, bees are becoming a memory of childhood for most adults.

It is against this backdrop that the threat to Hope Clinic and our home became alarmingly real. Mr AJ, the new owner, could not be pacified. He was determined to go ahead with his plans. Locals and patrons of Hope would have to resort to numerous passive resistance methods including obstructing attempts at excavation. One such effort involved laying down in the path of the bulldozers when they attempted a secret invasion at 3 am.

Mr. AJ was a church going man, who liked to boast about his financial support of his parish. We tried soft persuasion. We got the local Catholic Nuns to persuade him to abandon the quarry idea and cajole him into selling the land to us. In return I promised to create a small memorial garden in his Mother's memory in a corner of the property. We invited him for tea for a friendly discourse. He proposed that we sell our property including our home and clinic to him. He offered us an excellent price so that he could have more land for his proposed quarry!

The tug of war continued for three years. Over time, he succeeded in obtaining so called "sanctions" to dig on multiple occasions. Each time, he was stopped in his tracks by trucks full of villagers and Hope Charity patrons who showed up at the collector's office to obtain more "stays" suspending all activities. At the end of three years, AJ finally gave up and agreed to sell the land. Unintentionally, and through no planning on my part, I had become responsible for another 3.5 acres of land in India, where I had spent barely a month every year. The reason for this chain of events would become clear in the coming months.

A few years prior to that I went through a traumatic and enlightening experience of my son being diagnosed with a serious illness. He recovered from the illness after strong and toxic medications were used. Trained and practicing as an internist in the United States and well-versed in the nuances of the toxic effects of these drugs, I began to look into alternative health practices to detoxify my son so that he would not fall victim to negative consequences in the future. This quest led me to the ancient medicine practiced in India called Ayurveda.

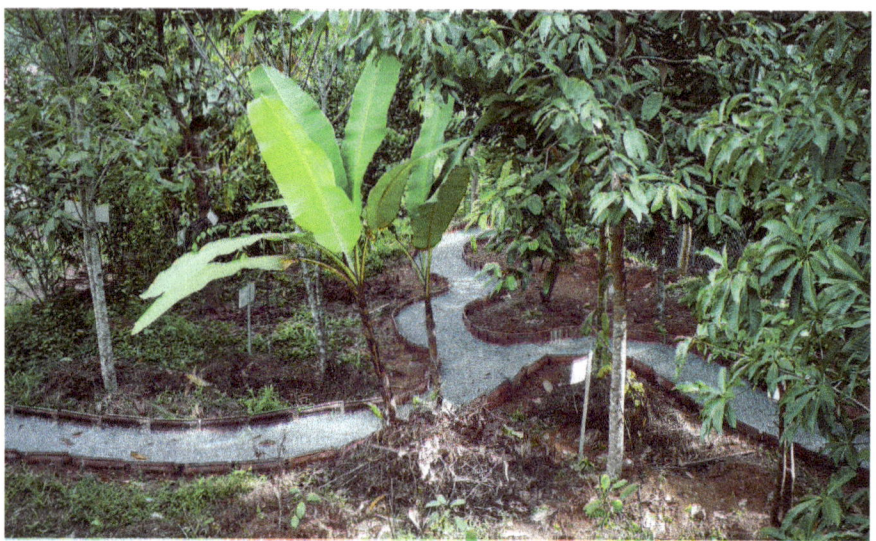

Ayurveda is a Sanskrit word that translates to "The Science of Life." It is a compilation of knowledge passed down through the ages. It is a guide to help humans live in maximum consciousness and awareness, by achieving optimal, physical, mental and spiritual health, all the while living in harmony with nature. When a human being falls out of balance or is ill with disease, the remedies can be found in this ancient system. They come from nature, flora and fauna and ones own body's healing mechanisms. With the looming threat of global warming, these plants are dying off one by one, risking the loss of healing knowledge permanently.

A few weeks after we had purchased the land, one day, I woke from an afternoon nap, basking in the radiance of an epiphany that made the purpose of this land crystal clear to me. The land would become a museum to showcase some of the most commonly used plants in Ayurvedic Medicine, many of which are rare and endangered, including ancient trees. It would also grow ancient fruits and vegetables and rekindle the memory and knowledge of what existed and what is still possible.

That year when the Hope Volunteer students visited, I talked to Karl about how I was dreaming about an environmental sustainability project. Once again, synchronicity would perform its magic. While doing research regarding medicinal plants, I met yet another Dr. Sashi from the Kerala Forestry Service. Dr Sashi, an expert in Medicinal Plants and Rare and Endangered Trees, had 22 new species of plants named after him. I would need Dr. Shashi to visit the property and give me advice on how to proceed.

In the meantime, Mr. AJ had clear cut the land, most of which was covered with rubber trees. They left it bare except for a smattering of income-generating timber species which were present on the property for many years. He left the land pregnant with the menacing root systems of the rubber trees which could be up to twenty feet deep.

For two weeks the bulldozers worked from sunrise to dusk, extracting the tentacles of intertwined roots and left-over rubber tree trunks. The bulldozers then carved out terraces to create flat garden plots in the hillside. These terraces were for the various gardens I envisioned from my year of research and consultation with the experts. In a rush of inspiration and excitement, I had drawn a preliminary plan of the landscape in an eight-hour marathon session while on a fourteen-hour flight to Kerala from Los Angeles.

The bulldozers dug up orange-crimson loamy soil left thousands of years ago from the of volcanic eruptions grinding and churning. The remnants of a dormant volcano created the hill. The hollow lava rocks, like meditating giants across the hilltop, bore testimony to the cataclysmic events that engendered the unmatched fertility of the soil's biodiversity. Finally, the land was ready to welcome its new occupants.

The rain showers arrived a few weeks later, soaking the dormant buried seeds which were now dug up into the surface soil. Within a week, the newly prepared land was blanketed by a lush green spray of new vegetation.

Dr Sashi visited a few months later. By this time, the brush covering the land was several feet tall. Dr. Sashi was a quiet, unassuming person and a man of few words. He was still in mourning for the loss his daughter to a fatal illness. Although we had not met before and had only a few conversations on the phone, he proceeded straight up the path and up to the hilltop as soon as he arrived. His black leather dress shoes were covered in a coat of orange-red dust by the time he reached the top. He was single minded and focused. Without a word, his camera appeared from his pocket. He began snapping photos of the fauna that interested him. He scanned the lay of the land and the garden plots. He squatted briefly and grabbed a fist full of the soil, rubbing it between his fingers. I was afraid to interrupt his silence. I did not want to interrupt his train of thought. After an hour we headed back. On the way back, he spotted a patch with many plants that seemed to hold him in one place for several minutes.

Finally, Dr. Sashi allowed himself to speak. He told me that there were close to ninety species of plants that he counted on the property, which are on the verge of extinction. He then cordoned off a small patch of vegetation towards the lower part of the garden with a red ribbon, asking us not to touch it as he was interested in discovering what would grow naturally on the land once the rubber trees were removed. He also promised to supply me with the plants needed for planting in a garden representing common medicinal plant species and Rare and Endangered Trees (RET). That year I visited various Agricultural Universities in Northern Kerala including KFRI (Kerala Forest Research Institute) and Botanical Gardens throughout Kerala.

In September of 2012, the saplings arrived. The planting was completed over two hot humid days into the thirsty parched soil. We prayed for rain and, four hours after planting was completed, the skies opened and baptized Ahimsa with a thunderous, downpour from the generous skies. The word Ahimsa means "non-violence", towards oneself and others. The Ahimsa Garden was born!

The sun has now risen and set over this patch of land close to 2600 times, and imparted growth, birth and death, all bringing forth to what the universe wills into existence. Many trees have grown to immense heights of over sixty feet, many have grown slowly and deliberately choosing to sculpt themselves into shapes and shades of their own choosing, many stand maimed, with dry limbs sticking out, resurrecting themselves with every rain. Many have withered and returned to the soil. Shrubs and vines reduced to brittle twigs snap and scatter in the scorching heat of summer to appear yet again with the next rain, flowering and bearing fruits. The garden continues to pick itself up after each scorching summer and draught, springing up within days with the slightest cloudburst that arrives eventually. Species that we did not plant, which were buried below the rubber trees, have emerged.

The wisdom of humility and submission has taken hold after the initial years of choreographing and cultivating. The wisdom that begets the courage to weave meaningful fulfillment and joy from strands of loss, disappointment and sorrow. The wisdom that keeps one sipping from every last drop of beauty and delight that the Universe bestows every moment. The wisdom that molds the unshaken faith that gives birth to the brutal optimism to carry on. The wisdom that above all teaches us to concentrate on duty, disconnecting oneself from the pleasure and pain of the results.

I sit on the verandah at dawn, the seventh year after the garden's beginning, writing these words. The curtains are raised and the play of nature is in full swing. Birds chime in one by one until the melodies are interrupted by the cacophony of crows, demanding attention. The last sliver of moon before the new moon arrives is still shining in the eastern sky amidst the stubborn stars that resist fading. Dawn paints the silhouettes of trees against the brightening canvas of the morning skies. While the sun, adorned in its fiery cloak, floats up hidden toward the horizon, prepared to manifest another day of miracles, making energies dance to create and destroy.

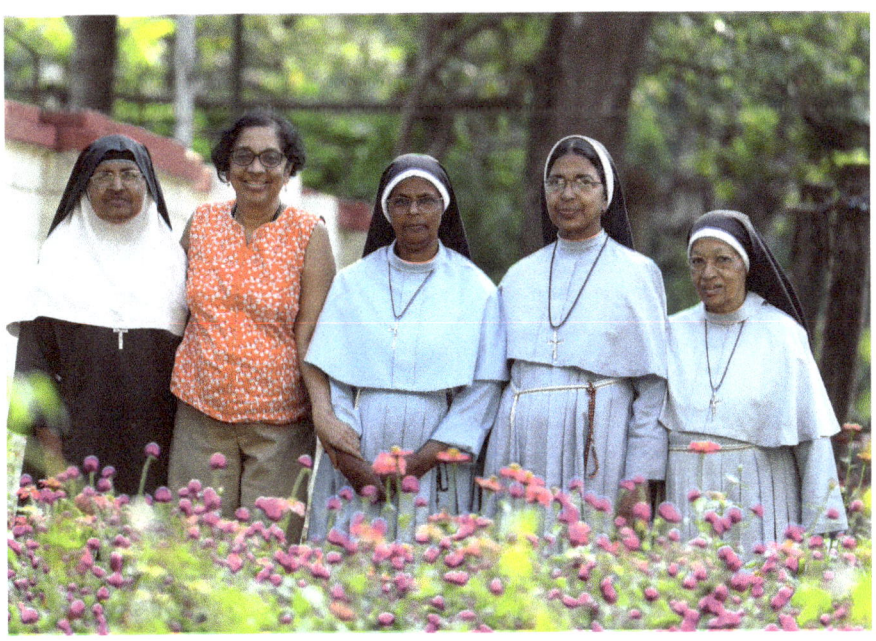

Author with nuns whose prayers and encouragement keep the project alive

THE SPICE WHEEL
The Basics of Use of Spices in Indian Cooking

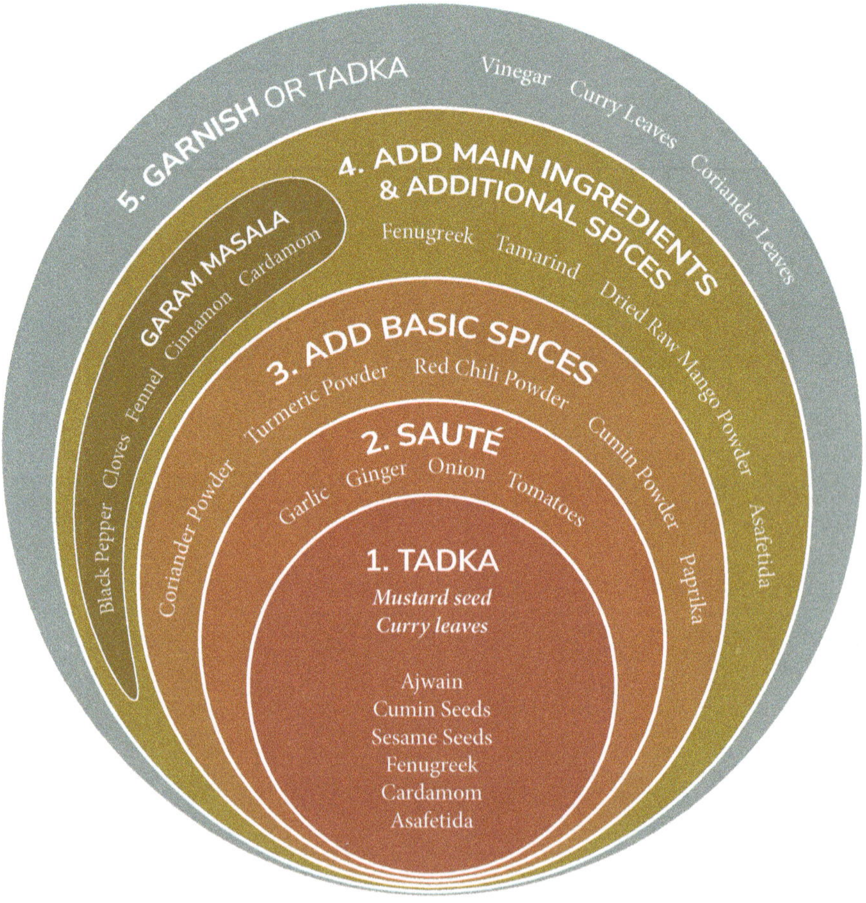

5. GARNISH OR TADKA
Vinegar, Curry Leaves, Coriander Leaves

4. ADD MAIN INGREDIENTS & ADDITIONAL SPICES
Fenugreek, Tamarind, Dried Raw Mango Powder, Asafetida, Paprika

GARAM MASALA
Black Pepper, Cloves, Fennel, Cinnamon, Cardamom

3. ADD BASIC SPICES
Coriander Powder, Turmeric Powder, Red Chili Powder, Cumin Powder

2. SAUTÉ
Garlic, Ginger, Onion, Tomatoes

1. TADKA
Mustard seed
Curry leaves

Ajwain
Cumin Seeds
Sesame Seeds
Fenugreek
Cardamom
Asafetida

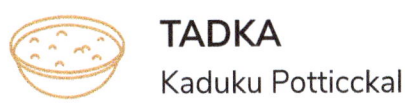

TADKA
Kaduku Potticckal

TADKA is a common cooking procedure that takes place at the beginning or end of the preparation of many Indian dishes.

The spice Wheel on the left is a depiction of how spices are added in the different stages of TADKA and cooking. **TADKA might take place in circle 1 or 5 and ingredients are proportionately selected from the group in each circle based on the dish.**

TADKA PROCESS

- Heat 1-3 tsp of oil of choice.
- When recipes require that TADKA be done at the **beginning** of the cooking, place mustard seeds and/or one or more of the ingredients from circle 1 into the oil and stir gently until brown.
- With mustard seeds one has to follow a special procedure. After the mustard seeds are put into hot oil, within 1 to 20 seconds, the mustard seeds will begin to pop. It is important to keep the pan partially covered or covered with a mesh lid to prevent the seeds from popping out on to the counter. One has to take caution to keep a slight distance from the popping seeds for personal safety.
- If TADKA is done at the **end** of cooking, follow the process above and pour contents of the pan over the fully cooked dish.

A significant number of Indian Recipes follow this general sequence outlined:

TADKA → SAUTÉ → ADD BASIC SPICES → ADD MAIN INGREDIENT & ADDITIONAL SPICES → GARNISH/TADKA

GLOSSARY

- *Asafetida*
  Gum oleoresin-pungent herb reminiscent of onion and leek used since Ancient Greek and Roman times. Reduces gas and bloating when cooked in lentil or vegetarian dishes.

- *Ayurveda*
  Ancient Indian system of medicine and wellbeing.

- *BMI*
  BMI or Body Mass Index is a ratio of height to weight that is used to determine whether or not an individual is maintaining a healthy weight.

- *Caste System (Indian)*
  Ancient system of social, economic, ethnic and class segregation and stratification based on the family and community an Indian is born into.

- *Factory Farm*
  Large scale and high environmental impact industrial farm with large turnover.

- *Gut Flora*
  Microorganisms in the gut that help our bodies digest and extract nutrients from food.

- *Kerala*
  A southwestern province of India

- *Kerala Backwaters*
  The Louisiana Bayou of India. The people of this area are traditional, rural and deeply Roman Catholic and earn their living by tilling the soil and fishing the local waters,

- *Malabar*
  Geographic and cultural region of SW India. The rural way of life in this area is shaped by the Arabian Sea and Western Ghats mountains that surround it on both sides.

- *Masala*
  Spice mixes made to season different dishes

- *Mumbai (Bombay)*
  Most populous city in India. One of the world's most historically and culturally rich cities located along the Arabian Sea and with

thriving entertainment, industrial and financial industries.

- *Pooja*
Ancient yet still widely practiced Hindu worship ritual. Performed as an everyday practice as well as a part of important events such as marriage, exams, moving to a new home, etc.

- *Probiotics*
Living microorganisms that are essential to human health due to their fueling of the digestive system.

- *Sattvic Diet*
Combinations of food that when consumed increases the quality and quantity of life

- *Toddy*
Traditional palm wine derived from coconut palm and a major part of Keralan society, culture, cuisine, politics, history and economy.

- *Yoga*
Practice originating in Ancient India with the goal of maintenance of physical, mental and spiritual health.

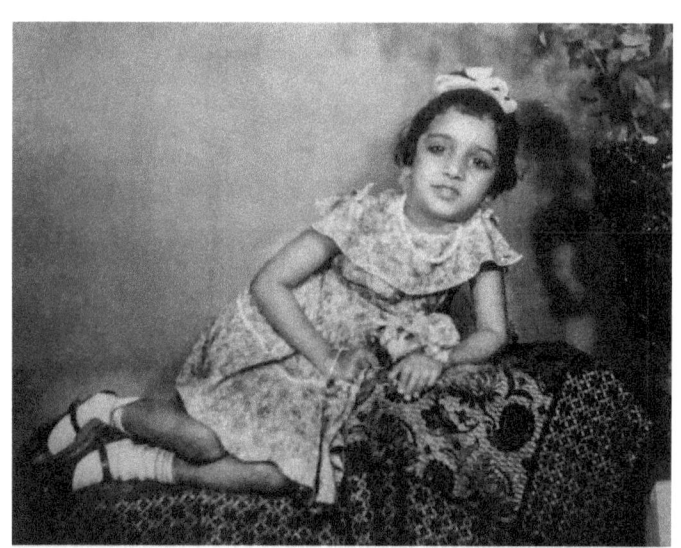

Author at age 4 in Kerala

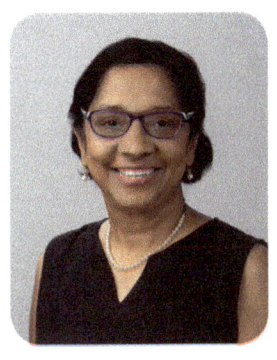
Dr. Daisy Kuchinad is a non-conformist physician in the US who practices medicine on her own terms. She is board certified in the Western allopathic disciplines of Internal Medicine and Geriatrics and has practiced Western medicine for over thirty years. Dissatisfied with Western medicine alone, she sought out and immersed herself in understanding Ayurveda, the ancient medical science of India. She believes in facilitating healing through an integrative approach, uniting Western mechanistic science and Eastern systems-based science with a goal of addressing root causes of disease. In 2001, she founded Hope Charities, Inc. (now BIRDS), which served over 2500 people with outpatient medical care and offered educational scholarships to low-income youth. In 2014, she started Ahimsa Retreats in Kerala, India, which provides Ayurveda, yoga, and meditation for groups from all over the world. Presently, she has started her own integrative medicine consultation practice in the US where she borrows from both modern allopathic and ancient Ayurvedic principles to more effectively address health issues at their core.

www.ingramcontent.com/pod-product-compliance
Lightning Source LLC
Chambersburg PA
CBHW061231070526
44584CB00030B/4074